The Cardiovascular Cure

The

Cardiovascular

Cure

How to Strengthen Your Self-Defense
Against Heart Attack and Stroke

John P. Cooke, M.D., Ph.D.,

and Judith Zimmer

BROADWAY BOOKS

NEW YORK

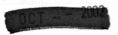

Library of Congress Cataloging-in-Publication Data
Cooke, John P.
The cardiovascular cure : how to strengthen your self-defense against heart attack and stroke / John P. Cooke and Judith Zimmer.
p. cm.
Includes index.
1. Cardiovascular system—Diseases—Popular works. 2. Cardiovascular system—Diseases—Prevention. 3. Nitric oxide—Physiological effect. 4. Vascular endothelium. I. Zimmer, Judith. II. Title.
RC672.C625 2002
616.1'05—dc21
2001055369

FIRST EDITION

Designed by JoAnne Metsch

ISBN 0-7679-0881-3

10 9 8 7 6 5 4 3 2 1

Contents

Acknowledgments

STANDING ON the shoulders of giants, one can see farther. For their past mentorship and guidance I am grateful to Drs. John T. Shepherd and Paul Vanhoutte at the Mayo Clinic, who introduced me to the endothelium, and Dr. Victor J. Dzau at Harvard, who showed me how to survive in academic medicine.

Scientific discovery is a community enterprise, and in this community I have many valued colleagues who have collaborated with me, including Drs. Edward Alderman, Robert Balint, Judith Berliner, Dan Bernstein, Margaret Billingham, Nanette Bishopric, Peter Black, Terry Blaschke, Dan Bloch, Eugene Butcher, Mark Creager, Myron Cybulsky, Peter Davies, John Deanfield, Helmut Drexler, Prakash Deedwania, Aldona Dembinska-Kiec, Mary and Marguerite Engler, Louis Fajardo, John Fallon, Gary Fathman, Peter Fitzgerald, Nick Flavahan, Michael Fowler, Peter Ganz, Gary Gibbons, Scott Herron, Mark Hlatky, Brian Hoffman, Don Houston, Bob Hu, Lou Ignarro, Tsutomo Imaizumi, Fran Johnson, Masumi Kimoto, John Kosek, Larry Leung, Amir Lerman, Joe Loscalzo, Tom Luscher, Rene Malinow, Mike Mendelsohn, Ed Mocarski, Ruichi Morishita, Randy Morris, Bill Parmley, Richard Pratt, Gerry Reaven, Tom Rimele, Bobby Robbins, Jonathan Rothbard, Gabor Rubanyi, Angelo Scuteri, Jonathan Stamler, Thomas Quertermous, Hannah Valantine, Patrick Vallance, Sir John Vane, and Alan Yeung.

Much of the credit for the scientific foundation of this book is due the young scientists and research assistants who have worked with me. These are bright and dedicated individuals from every corner of the globe who have engaged me with their imagination and energy: Drs. Vinod Achan, Shanthi Adimoolam, Susan Alpert, Nancy Andon, Mehrdad Arjomandi, Stephanie Bode-Boger, Rainer Boger, Ricardo Buitrago, Robert Candipan, Jason Chan, Henry Chen, Jaw-Wen Chen, Jenny Chen, Hayan Dayoub, Dan Dubin, Josef Dulak, Bill Fearon, Guy Haywood, Xavier Girerd, Chris Heeschen, Hoai-Ky Vu Ho, Paul Hsiun, Akira Ito, Johannes Jacobi, James Jang, Shariar Heidari, Bob Kernoff, Subbu Lakshmi, Lynette Lissin, Neil Lewis, Kenny Lin, Patrick Lin, Pia Lundman, Adrian Ma, Andy Maxwell, Leslie McEvoy, Joseph Neibauer, Minoru Ohno, Roberta Oka, Matt Pollman, Gene Rossitch, A. C. Santosa, Severin Schwarzacher, Alan Singer, Markus Stuehlinger, Andrzej Szuba, Phil Tsao, Gregor Theilmeier, Shiro Uemura, Heiko von der Leyen, Bing-Yin Wang, Yan Wang, Michael Ward, Franz Weidinger, Michael Weis, Andreas Wolf, and Christof Zalpour.

Medicine is an art, and as one of the newest disciplines, vascular medicine is a work in progress. Fellow artisans who have labored with me in defining this new field include Drs. Lucien Abenhaim, John Callahan, Trip Casscells, Mariella Catalano, Denis Clement, Les Cooper, Jack Farquhar, Ed Frohlich, Bill Haskell, Bill Hiatt, Alan Hirsch, Jeff Isner, Iain Johnston, John Joyce, Janice Marshall, Lars Norgren, Jeff Olin, Judy Regensteiner, Bob Safford, Jack Spittell, Saskia Thiadens, and Jon Tooke.

The work can't get done without people who assist with the administrative details of basic and clinical research, manuscripts, and funding, and so I thank Gabriella Bakonyi, Ritu Bhatnagar, Om Kapoor, Kirsten Leute, Liz Lopez, Scott Reiff, Azadeh Soltani, Paige Stefik, Ruth Graves, Mary Watanabe, and Shuja Yousuf. To Luigi and Pisana Deciani, I treasure the time I spent at your villa nestled in the foothills of the Italian Alps where I was inspired to draft the final chapters of the book.

For believing in the ideas, and putting significant effort and/or funding into developing my ideas into useful products that help people with heart disease, I am most grateful to Moshe and Hannah Ariel, John Giannuzzi, Kenny Pettine, Martine Rothblatt, and Darlene Walley. I am also grateful for the support of Bruce and Duane Abbott, Barb Anderson, The Angel's Forum, Lisa Marie Aeschlimann, Josef Ariel, Asahi Breweries, Paul Auerbach, Bruce Benedict, Robert Bjorn,

Mark Bonham, Adam Borison, Arnold Breit, Roger Brooks, Kristen Bruinsma, Peter and Joyce Burfield, Douglas and Cloy Burnett, Adam Newman Burton, Chuck Calalano, the Capulong family, Robert Carbonell, Mark Carey, James and Kuang Chang, Frances Cohen, Michael Compton, Lauren Cooks and Paul Levitan, Anna and Patrick Cooke, Joseph Cooper, Ron Corran, George Croom, Michael Crady, Elizbeth Dailey, Jon D'Alessio, Shannon Denson, William Dieters, Jurgen Dominik, Jay Eisenlohr, Robert Epstein, John Fara, Arthur Ferrara, Tim Fischell, Lloyd Flanders, Thomas Fogarty, David Garcia, Bill Gatti, General Mills, Robert Gries, Ken Griffith, Peter Gumina, Donald and Sue Ann Hansen, Scott Hanson, William and Helen Hawkins, Donald Hejna, Ralph Hirsch, Hitachi Ltd., Joseph Hudson, Itochu Corp., J&J Venture Fund, Norman Jangaard, Chen Jong, Tjandra Kahar, Christine Kenworthy, Fahir Kirdar, Frank Koch, Peter and Marilee Kovacs, Lester and Patricia Krupp, Mary Anne LaHaye, Jing Lapus, Robert Levinsky, Lombard-Odier, Martin Lowenstein, Deanna Minich, Abraham Nader, Senator Ernesto Maceda (Philippines), Gary and Barbara Martinelli, Samuel Marty, Walter and Mary McCullough, Mead Johnson, Craig and Natalie Miller, Georgio Moro, Erika Lynn Moses, Putra Mosagung, Ben Muhlenkamp and Nellson Nutriceutical, Robert Mullis and Kimberley Nadeau, New Medical Technologies, the Newman family, Ruediger Noumann-Etienne, Roderik and Sylvia O'Reilly, John Onoboni, Phillip Pace, Araceli Panaligan, Fred Pashkow, David Paul, Eve Pearl, James Peterson, Edwin Perez, Russell and Sally Porter, Michael Rabson, Phillip Raiser, Robin Robinson, Mariles Romulo, John J. Rose, Jay Rosenfeld, Bert Rowland, Wilfred and Marianna Samson, John Sanguinetti, Edmund Shamsi, Michael Schwartzman, Sabrina Schulz, Francis Scott and Patricia Smyth, Luanna Shaughnessy, Michael Silbert, Joel Sklar, Norman Sokiloff, the Songcayawons, Stanford University, Dr. Fred St. Goar, Wes Sterman, John and Marsha Stevens, Spencer and Mary Tall, Ben Trainer, Robert Tomasello, Steven Tuch, Don Tyson, Joel Uchenik, Jr., Paul Ulrich, Manny Villar, Thadeus Vogler, Paul and Dorothy Wachter, Vandita Wilson, Warren Wong, Paul and Cynthia Yock, Kenneth Yip, Michael Zapien, and Norma Zimmer.

This book would not have come to fruition without the help of Angela Miller, who guided me through the publishing world and brought me into contact with Judith Zimmer, who is a terrific medical writer. Jennifer Josephy, my editor, has great vision and a skillful touch. Dana Jacobi formulated, tested, and refined the recipes in the book with great skill. And finally, Judith Zimmer and I want to acknowledge our spouses (Alastair Standing and Robin Cooke), who gave us great support during the climb to the summit!

Special thanks to Ann Coulston, MS, RD, FADA, and former president of the American Dietetic Association, for her guidance in developing the nutritional recommendations in this book.

Foreword

I HAVE BEEN immersed in biological research for more than half a century, and in 1982, received the Nobel Prize for my discovery of a prostaglandin that we called prostacyclin. It relaxes blood vessels, a property that has led to new treatments for heart and vessel disease. I was also cited for discovering the way that aspirin and similar drugs work, again through interactions with the prostaglandin system.

I have had the great pleasure of exchanging ideas with bright and innovative investigators the world over. When I first met John Cooke some years ago in his laboratory at Stanford University, he struck me as an enthusiastic young clinical scientist with great promise. His subsequent research work and the publication of this book show how right I was!

Over the last 50 years biologists have discovered many different mediators or chemical messengers, which transmit signals from one cell to another. They include amines such as histamine, acetylcholine, and catecholamines; peptides such as bradykinin and angiotensin; and lipids such as prostacyclin. They all play important roles in keeping the body working, and because of this, Nobel Prizes have been awarded to several of the discoverers. Less than 15 years ago, a different and very potent mediator of blood vessel relaxation and inhibition of platelet clumping was identified as nitric oxide (NO). It is the simplest messenger of them all, and as a gas, will diffuse freely through cell membranes.

This gas, a one-to-one combination of the two main elements of the air, nitrogen and oxygen, was, until then, recognized only as a toxic pollutant in the exhausts of cars or as a product formed in the atmosphere as the result of thunder and lightning flashes. However, in the last two decades we have learnt, through the research work of scientists such as John Cooke, that NO is formed in the body to help maintain the health of the blood vessels and the heart. There are special enzymes that generate NO from arginine (an amino acid contained in our food), and we now know it has important functions in the brain, the immune system, and the vasculature.

As a Nobel laureate, I sometimes go to Stockholm to participate in the yearly prize ceremony on the anniversary of Alfred Nobel's death on December 10. In 1998, I had the privilege of seeing the prize in Physiology or Medicine awarded to three Americans, Bob Furchgott, Lou Ignarro, and Ferid Murad, for their "discoveries concerning nitric oxide as a signalling molecule in the cardiovascular system." It was a glorious occasion when the scientific and medical world honored the leaders of research on this most important molecule, which plays a pivotal part in the health of our circulation.

John Cooke has made his own brilliant contribution to what we know about the endothelial lining of our blood vessels and the part that NO plays in keeping it healthy. But he has done more than that. He has thought deeply about the ways that we can rearrange our diet in order to maximize the production of nitric oxide. He has carefully and methodically searched for foods that contain arginine and has also brought his scientific prowess to examining other aspects of a healthy diet. He has invented an arginine-enriched medical food as a convenient way of supplying arginine (and other vascular nutrients) to those who need it.

But this is much more than just another book about dietary fads. It is the first diet I have seen that bases the recommended menus and recipes on proven scientific facts. More than that, it is eminently readable and avoids the clumsy use of unexplained scientific jargon. I am sure that you will enjoy reading it (and following the diet!) as much as I have.

SIR JOHN VANE, D.SC., F.R.S.
NOBEL LAUREATE, 1982
Honorary President, William Harvey Research Foundation
Professor of Pharmacology, William Harvey Research Institute
London, England
November 2001

Introduction

You are only as old as your endothelium.

—PAUL VANHOUTTE, *Mayo Clinic (1983)*

THERE IS magic within us. It is a magic that arises from the genetic code, taking form within the complex interaction between cells and tissue. It is a magic that can lengthen your life, a magic that can be strengthened or weakened depending on how you nourish it. What you do with the magic is up to you.

This book will introduce you to the magic that is inside your blood vessels. It comes in the shape of a molecule, one of the simplest molecules found in nature. This molecule is nitric oxide, or NO, a substance so powerful that it can actually protect you from heart attack and stroke. Best of all, your body can make it on its own. NO is your body's own built-in, natural protection against heart disease.

Today, thanks to new research in cardiovascular medicine, we know much more about blood vessels than we did just a few years ago. In fact, we now know that cardiovascular disease affects not only the heart, but also the miles of blood vessels throughout the body. We know that blood vessels are more than passive pipes that get blocked. We also know much more about atherosclerosis, or hardening of the arteries, the disease of the blood vessels that results in heart attack and stroke and is the number one cause of death in this country.

We now recognize that the inflammatory process plays an important role in the buildup of plaque. And that this buildup is more than deposits in a pipe that need to be mechanically removed, dilated with a balloon, or bypassed surgically.

This book will introduce you to this new concept in vascular medicine. The body is capable of healing itself. Damaged and blocked vessels can open up and function normally again.

When I was in medical school in the mid-1980s, we were taught that atherosclerosis was an end-stage condition, a disease that everyone would get as they grew older. But that's just not true. We now know that we have a choice regarding this disease. With a diet and lifestyle that channels the natural forces of the blood vessel, atherosclerosis can be prevented, brought to a halt, and even reversed.

You can take care of your blood vessels, just as you can take care of other parts of your body. Blood vessels are alive and vital like any other organ in the body. They can change their diameter and control the blood flow through them. You have 100,000 miles of blood vessels in a complex network throughout your body. A roadblock anywhere can lead to a serious medical problem, such as debilitating leg pain, stroke, or heart attack.

If you haven't given much thought to blood vessel health until now, you're not alone. Most internists, and even cardiologists, know very little about blood vessels and vascular disease. (There are only about a dozen medical schools in the U.S. where vascular medicine is taught.) Instead, physicians trained in cardiovascular medicine spend most of their time concentrating on the heart as a pump. Many cardiologists are focused on catheter-based interventions, performing angioplasties and putting in stents. These can be useful procedures in certain situations. But I think that there is too much emphasis on technology to get rid of symptoms and not enough focus on strengthening the body's own healing process.

My cardiac specialization has been in vascular medicine—concentrating on the function and health of blood vessels. Physicians in vascular medicine conduct research in, and take care of patients with, vascular disorders. We are interested in how blood vessels control the flow of blood; how they keep the blood from clotting; how vessels prevent their walls from thickening. We study the processes that lead to blockages in vessels and how these blockages can be prevented.

As director of vascular medicine at Stanford University, I run one of the first NIH-created centers for vascular medicine. Stanford has a history of excellence in this field. Heart transplantation in the U.S. originated here and many high-tech devices were created here to both detect and treat heart disease. In addition, there is an honorable tradition of research in disease prevention. In that tradition, I conduct research, see patients in our Vascular Medicine Clinic, and teach the use of diet and lifestyle changes to improve the health of blood vessels.

In the course of the last few years, we have learned some surprising new things in our study of blood vessels and through our care of people with heart and vessel disease. This new knowledge may save your life. I am convinced that if you use the knowledge in this book, you will live a longer and healthier life.

Say Yes to NO (Nitric Oxide)

ONE OF the most exciting new findings in cardiovascular medicine involves the molecule nitric oxide, or NO. We now know that our bodies produce nitric oxide in the endothelium (pronounced en-do-theel-e-um), a delicate tissue that is the inner lining of the blood vessel. The endothelium is so significant to blood vessel health that I predict that in the next few years the health of your endothelium will become as important as cholesterol to you and your doctor.

In 1998, three American researchers won the Nobel Prize in Medicine for their discoveries concerning NO in the cardiovascular system. (One of the researchers named it EDRF, which stands for endothelium-derived relaxing factor; the two names—EDRF and NO—refer to the same thing.) Previously believed to be a hazardous air pollutant outside the body, nitric oxide was found to provide a host of benefits inside the body. Nitric oxide was hailed as an important molecule not only in the field of cardiovascular medicine but also in many medical disciplines, including infectious medicine, pulmonary medicine, and oncology. (As early as 1992, *Science* magazine named it the "molecule of the year," based on the incredible amount of evidence pointing to its importance in the healthy function of our bodies.)

The discovery of nitric oxide had a great impact on the world of cardiovascular medicine. We learned that the endothelium was much more than it seemed. It was the proverbial "silver" lining. The endothelium creates NO, its own heart medicine!

The way NO works is simple yet revolutionary. Its power is due, in part, to the fact that it is 100 percent natural. Healthy individuals produce NO in their blood vessels. The healthier you are, the more NO you make.

You are probably, and rightly, wondering, If NO is so potent and so protective, then why is there so much heart and vessel disease in this country? Unfortunately, most Americans are not producing enough NO in their blood vessels. Why not? Because many people have high blood pressure or high levels of cholesterol, sugar, and fat in their blood. They may smoke. These people all make less NO. And finally, there is a risk factor that we are all susceptible to—aging. Unfortunately, in many people, these risk factors begin a downhill course that leads to reduced vitality, less ability to exercise, and eventually symptoms of heart and vascular disease.

But the good news is that the human body is remarkably restorative (and forgiving) when it comes to vascular health. In my lab at Stanford and others around the country, we are learning about how to restore the body's production of NO and to harness its power for vascular and heart health.

Heart Disease—the Number One Killer

DURING MY years as a physician/scientist at the Mayo Clinic, Harvard Medical School, and the Stanford University School of Medicine, I have seen firsthand the toll that cardiovascular disease takes on Americans and people in other industrialized countries around the world. For example:

- The Boston judge, known for the eloquence and clarity of his carefully crafted legal opinions, reduced to helplessness by a stroke that left his speech unintelligible, his face distorted, and his left side paralyzed.

- The Minnesota farmer who ignored the pressure in his chest as he baled hay. He came to the emergency room only after the crops were in. He was pale, sweaty, and short of breath—and had a massive heart attack that left him permanently weakened and unable to withstand the rigors of farming.

- The Long Island housewife who could not give up smoking, even though blood flow to her left leg had slowed to a trickle, causing constant foot pain and gangrene in her toes.

The list of people goes on and on. I've seen so much suffering, so many good years cut short, so many productive individuals crippled, so many families saddled with medical bills. To me, this is all the more tragic because the suffering and the limitations could have been forestalled, and even prevented entirely.

Let's face it: we all need to take better care of our heart and blood vessels. Just look at the obituaries for a few days for a jolt of reality. Most deaths in the United States and Europe (and increasingly in Asia) are due to heart attack and stroke—and about 30 percent of these unfortunate people are in their 50s and 60s. Today, the average age of our population is about 35, according to *Age: 2000,* a publication of the U.S. Census Bureau. Although many of us in this age bracket would like to ignore the possibility of dying from cardiovascular disease, we simply cannot. We all need to take better care of our cardiovascular health. As we get older, our risks for heart disease increase; this is true for women as well as men.

We now know that the health of the endothelium and the blood vessels directly affects overall cardiovascular health. Cardiovascular disease kills 500,000 Americans every year in the form of heart attack and stroke.[1] About 16 million more Americans suffer pain and disabilities caused by cardiovascular disease.

Today more than 60,800,000 Americans (a quarter of the U.S. population) have one or more conditions that put them at risk for heart attack and stroke! Cardiovascular disease—hypertension, coronary heart disease, heart failure, stroke, or peripheral arterial disease—has been the number one killer in the United States for over 80 years. One in five adults has some form of cardiovascular disease, and many more can expect to develop some form of the disease before age 60. The same grim statistics affect Europe. In Asia, cardiovascular disease is becoming more common as more people eat a Western-style diet and continue to smoke.

Stroke is a form of cardiovascular disease that blocks vessels supplying blood to the brain. Stroke, the leading cause of long-term disability in the U.S., kills about 160,000 Americans every year and is the third-leading cause of death, behind heart disease and cancer. (In Japan, it is the major cause of cardiovascular death.)

In an attempt to relieve chest pain, cardiologists in the U.S. perform more than 900,000 angioplasties annually, including 539,000 to open up diseased heart arteries. To prevent stroke, surgeons perform approximately 121,000 carotid endarterectomies (a procedure in which the surgeon scrapes plaque from the major arteries to the brain) annually.

Atherosclerosis can also affect the vessels that supply the legs with blood. Hardening of the leg arteries, known as peripheral arterial disease (PAD), causes aching of the legs while walking and, in its more severe manifestations, foot pain at rest, even gangrene. The most underdiagnosed vascular disease, PAD is believed to affect about 9 million Americans, most of whom don't realize they have the disease.

Atherosclerosis, which also affects blood flow to the pelvis and sexual organs, can cause impotence. In fact, the most common cause of impotence is "vasculogenic impotence," the inability to have or maintain an erection because of poor blood flow to the penis. A common feature of vasculogenic impotence is the inability to produce enough NO.

The economic costs of these vessel diseases are staggering. In 2001, the economic cost of all cardiovascular disease was approximately $298 billion, including health expenditures and lost productivity. Approximately 11 percent of these expenditures were for medication; over $27 billion was spent on cardiovascular drugs in 1998. The human costs are more difficult to estimate. Those of us with relatives or friends with the disease, and physicians who treat these patients, have witnessed its tragic consequences.

But it doesn't have to be this way.

Creating the Nutritional Program

WHEN I'M not treating patients, I'm in the lab, conducting research that seeks to understand the processes that lead to heart attack and stroke. To this end, I have been involved for the past 20 years in clinical practice and research at the Mayo Clinic, Harvard, and Stanford. At each institution, my research protocols were designed to find out what makes blood vessels healthy. From the beginning, my research has focused on the endothelium and its role in the structure, function, and behavior of the cardiovascular system.

We now know that a healthy endothelium produces NO, a substance responsible for a host of benefits in the blood vessel—increasing blood flow, preventing fatty deposits from sticking to the vessel wall, inhibiting thickening of the vessel wall, and reducing the chances of blood vessels constricting. If you have a healthy endothelium, the lining of your blood vessels is like Teflon, a smooth, nonstick surface that enhances the flow of blood. By contrast, if your endothelium is unhealthy, it is more like Velcro, causing white blood cells and platelets to stick to it.

Another important piece of the research puzzle was the discovery, by Dr. Salvador Moncada from England, that the endothelium uses the amino acid L-arginine to make nitric oxide. When that discovery was made, I was an assistant professor of medicine at Harvard Medical School directing my own lab. We had found that high levels of cholesterol impair the ability of the blood vessels to dilate. Based on Dr. Moncada's work, we experimented with L-arginine to see if it could increase the production of NO—and we were the first research group to show that additional L-arginine could restore the ability of the blood vessels to dilate. My research group, and others around the world, soon found that L-arginine could improve the blood vessel health of people with high cholesterol or vascular disease.

Since that time, we have learned much more from the work of many excellent scientists about specific changes in nutrition, lifestyle, and medication (if necessary) that can restore endothelial healh. This knowledge is so new that it has not been used in a systematic way until now. Building on what we have learned about the endothelium and how it can be enhanced by diet, exercise, and nutritional supplements, I have created a program for endothelial health. Its foundation is my research at Stanford and the work of many other scientists. This powerful new diet and lifestyle program is specifically designed to make your blood vessels and your endothelium healthier and to stimulate NO production and to enhance its activity. I am currently treating patients with this program and they are thriving—with relieved symptoms of angina and leg pain, renewed energy, better sex lives, and less risk of heart attack and stroke. And the benefits of the program can be felt in as little as two weeks!

This book is divided into three sections, designed to improve your understanding of vascular medicine and the health of your endothelium. In Part 1, you will learn about the discovery of nitric oxide and what that means for the health of your blood vessels. You will find out about new research in atherosclerosis and what we now know about plaque forming—and rupturing—within blood vessels. You will understand how this new research in cardiovascular medicine can help prevent, and reverse, atherosclerosis.

Part 2 will introduce you to my program for endothelial health. The three elements of the program include the diet, exercise, and dietary supplement recommendations. Here you will find new insights about keeping your blood vessels healthy with nutrition and exercise. To get you started, I have provided two weeks of menus and recipes.

Part 3 will help you to evaluate the health of your endothelium and to determine the intensity of the program you need. You will also learn more about dietary supplements that can reduce your risk factors and make you feel better. There is also an in-depth discussion of intensive care for the blood vessels for those who need it, with recommendations regarding medication.

If you or your physician want more information (or references) on these topics, I have supplied a section called Information for Your Doctor at the back of the book.

INTRODUCING THE DIET

AT THE heart of the endothelial health program is the diet, a baseline nutrition program for everyone. It features two weeks of menus that provide you with a pattern of healthy eating for a lifetime.

The diet is a carefully designed meal plan to help you maintain a healthy endothelium. It is a modification of the nutritional program of the well-known Lyon Diet Heart Study, conducted in France in the early 1990s. This study revealed that a Mediterranean-style diet (rich in polyunsaturated omega-3 fatty acids found in fish, nuts, and flaxseed oil) could reduce death and recurrent heart attack in patients with cardiovascular disease more than the standard American Heart Association diet. The benefits of this diet in reducing death from cardiovascular disease are similar to those of the most powerful lipid-lowering drugs! And, as you'll find, my diet goes even further than the Lyon diet in highlighting nutrients that benefit endothelial function.

My diet builds on the work that we have done at Stanford, as well as the work of many nutritionists, physicians, and researchers around the country. It is based on my personal experience, but also borrows from the best recommendations of the American Heart Association Nutrition Committee and other thoughtful leaders in cardiovascular medicine.

The diet features a balance of proteins rich in L-arginine, nutrient-dense carbohydrates, and healthy types of fat enriched with omega-3 fatty acids. It is designed to improve your lipid profile, maintain blood sugar and insulin in the normal range, and provide the key nutrients and vitamins needed for optimal blood vessel health—all in 1,800 calories a day.

While you will find many aspects of the diet to be familiar (intentionally so; we wanted to make the diet easy to follow), you will also find new ideas about soy and legumes, for example, foods that maximize your cardiovascular health. Realize that every food in our two-week menu plan has a direct beneficial effect on vascular health. You'll find recipes for easy-to-make delicious meals and desserts that will help you establish a healthy pattern of eating that can be continued for a lifetime.

I am often asked how it's possible to improve endothelial health in just two weeks. The endothelium is unusual in that its condition is very much affected by what you eat. Just one meal can hurt or help your endothelial health. So you can imagine the obvious benefit after two weeks of healthy meals! Obviously, the longer you are on the diet, the healthier your vessels will become.

The diet stands out for another reason—it is not a fad or trendy diet, but menu choices that are designed to instill a healthy eating pattern for life. This is the kind of diet that your own doctor will readily endorse.

EXERCISE PROGRAM

EXERCISE IS a crucial component of endothelial health. I encourage you, as I do all my patients, to embark on an exercise program, if you have not already done so. This book will help you to design an exercise program that is right for you. It is important to know what types of exercise are best for the health of your blood vessels.

We know that aerobic exercise increases blood flow through your vessels. The endothelium can sense this increase in flow and in response produce NO. Researchers know the type of exercise that is best for blood vessel health. They have found that people who participate in aerobic exercise—walking, jogging, swimming, or bicycling, for example—have improved endothelial health, regardless of their age.

NUTRIENTS, VITAMINS, AND DIETARY SUPPLEMENTS TO ENHANCE VESSEL HEALTH

WE HAVE learned a great deal in the last few years about how certain nutrients, vitamins, and dietary supplements can enhance the health of blood vessels. My diet takes advantage of this knowledge: the foods in our menus maximize vegetable and marine proteins rich in L-arginine; nutrient-dense carbohydrates from vegetables and fruits containing B vitamins and antioxidant phytochemicals; fiber; phytoestrogens; as well as healthy sources of fat, including monounsaturated, polyunsaturated, and omega-3 fatty acids.

In addition, there are other nutrients and vitamins that can be added to your diet, depending upon the health of your blood vessels. If you are at risk for developing heart disease or already have significant vessel damage, you need to know how you can strengthen your blood vessels with additional vitamins and supplements. This book will introduce you to the nutrients, vitamins, and supplements that I have successfully used to repair the functioning of the heart and blood vessels in many of my patients. You will learn a clear and methodical way to use these supplements to ensure that you get the most benefit from them. You will also gain the knowledge you need to be a discriminating shopper at the health food store or when shopping for supplements at the pharmacy.

How healthy is your endothelium? In Part 3, you will have a chance to answer that question, to find out about your own level of endothelial health and what you need to do to improve it.

There are several ways to measure endothelial function. So far, two companies have developed tests that measure endothelial health. Until these tests are widely distributed, risk factors for cardiovascular disease can also be used as a measure of endothelial health, since we know that the endothelium is not healthy if you have risk factors for heart disease.

Based on our Point System Risk Assessment test, you can determine your risk for cardiovascular disease. With your score in mind, you can follow one of three prescriptions for endothelial health.

• You are healthy, but concerned. So far, you are lucky—you have very few risks for heart disease. Still, you want to continue to maintain your vascular health at a high level. To do this, you must follow my diet and exercise program. This way, you'll maintain a healthy endothelium and protect yourself from cardiovascular disease.

• You have several risk factors for cardiovascular disease. The first and foremost priority for you is to lower your risk. I will explain how to do this and, in the process, show you how each risk factor impairs endothelial health. You will need to follow my diet and exercise program and use selected supplements or medications. In essence, this program will help you repair your endothelium.

· You have heart disease. Through my program, you will reduce the pain of angina or peripheral arterial disease and, in general, improve your cardiovascular health. You need to follow my diet, get clearance from a physician to pursue an exercise program, and take the vitamins and supplements that I recommend. Because you will also need medication, I will provide you with a "second opinion" on heart medications. I will also explain why I believe that too many Americans are turning to angioplasty as a solution to heart disease. Some of the angioplasties currently performed are utterly unnecessary (remember the unneeded cesarean sections and hysterectomies of the recent past). Although angioplasty may relieve symptoms, it does not reverse the disease the way our program of diet and lifestyle interventions can. In addition, angioplasty causes further damage to the vessel and completely destroys the delicate endothelial tissues. In about one-third of cases, this causes a wound-healing response in the vessels that leads to re-narrowing within three to six months. Although stents have reduced the frequency of this problem (and new drug-releasing stents do not cause much re-narrowing), no stent will reverse the process of atherosclerosis the way our program of dietary and lifestyle interventions can.

Reaping the Benefits of the Endothelium Health Program

MANY DOCTORS do not yet know about the new research in endothelial health or the benefits of a specialized dietary intervention to repair blood vessel damage. Nor are they adequately versed in the importance of the endothelium and its relationship to vascular disease. However, it has become increasingly clear to leading physicians and investigators that the key to reducing heart attack and stroke lies in restoring endothelial and vascular health.

Patients on my endothelial health program who previously suffered from angina and other symptoms of heart disease are living pain-free and report that the quality of their lives is much improved. Yours can be too!

To give you an idea of the kind of people who have benefited from my work, here is what happened to one of my patients, another physician at Stanford. Two years ago, when Dr. A. F. was 83, he thought he had to give up practicing medicine because his cardio-vascular health had deteriorated. A highly valued member of the Department of Medicine, Dr. A. F. could barely walk a half block before experiencing severe pain in his legs. And he had another worrisome problem—he had developed numbness in his left arm.

An astute clinician, Dr. A. F. of course knew what was wrong. He had developed the warning signs of atherosclerosis—specifically, narrowings in his leg and neck arteries. He had extensive tests that confirmed his fears; worse, the magnetic resonance images suggested that the smaller vessels in his brain were narrowed and that surgical correction of the brain arteries was not possible. He thought that there was nothing more that could be done, except to continue taking the medicine he was already taking. And he had a difficult decision to make. Because of the pain in his legs, he could no longer keep pace with the young doctors on hospital rounds. Moreover, he felt weighed down by the looming possibility of a stroke.

Dejected, Dr. A. F. prepared to resign and hang up his stethoscope after 60 years of being a doctor and teacher. A few days later, Dr. A. F. heard me talk at Medical Grand Rounds at Stanford about the work I was doing in restoring endothelial health. Dr. A. F. decided to try my program. Within a couple of weeks, he began to notice an improvement. The numbness in his arm went away and then disappeared completely. And he noticed that he could walk farther and farther—up to three blocks easily, enough to participate on rounds in the hospital.

Needless to say, everyone, including Dr. A. F., was pleased that he no longer had to quit doing what he loved. As I am writing this, the doctor is back on the wards at Stanford, doing what he loves best, healing and teaching.

Like Dr. A. F. and my other patients, you too will learn about the body's natural defense against heart attack and stroke. You will discover the steps you can take to enhance your body's natural defense mechanisms against atherosclerosis. No matter how old you are, or your current risk for heart disease, you can improve the condition of your cardiovascular system by following my endothelial health program. You will find that the benefits are both short- and long-term.

Within days of beginning the endothelium health program, your body's ability to make NO will improve dramatically. As a consequence, your blood vessels will become healthier and more relaxed.

Within as little as two weeks:

- You may experience less discomfort, if you have angina or other symptoms of heart disease.
- You will be able to walk farther and with less pain, if you have peripheral arterial disease (disease of the blood vessels of the leg).
- Your sexual vitality may be improved, if you have erectile dysfunction due to a vascular cause.

The reason you may see such a quick improvement in your health is that the endothelium can rapidly repair itself given the right ingredients. As endothelial health improves, the body is able to make more and more NO, thus improving the health of the blood vessels. The ability of the endothelium to rapidly recover has been documented by my research team, first at Harvard and later at Stanford. Our observations have been confirmed and extended by investigators at the best medical institutions worldwide.

These investigators and others have shown that NO activity is reduced in people with heart and vascular disease and that this impairment can be rapidly reversed with the diet, exercise, and supplement program prescribed in this book.

If, as I have explained, your endothelial health will improve within days of starting the program, imagine the long-term benefits. If you stay with my program for endothelial health and make it part of your lifestyle long-term, you will be continuously improving the structure and function of your blood vessels over time.

If you have hardening of the arteries (and most of us do), it has taken decades for these deposits to form. Any strategy designed to stabilize and shrink these deposits will take several years for maximum effect. If you adhere long-term to the basic elements of my endothelial health program, you will slow the progression of atherosclerosis and may even reverse its course.

With this book, I hope to bring this revolutionary new research and potentially life-saving information to those who most need it. Like the many patients I treat, each and every one of you has a different need when it comes to cardiovascular health. I have written this book so that you can gain new information about how to improve your current cardiovascular health. You are invited to take advantage of our website, www.cardiovascularcure.com.

When I was in training at the Mayo Clinic, one of my wise mentors, Paul Vanhoutte, was fond of saying, "You are only as old as your endothelium." Of course, he was right. Age is a determinant of endothelial function, but not the only one. I know 75-year-olds who have the endothelial function of 25-year-olds, and I have seen some 25-year-olds whose endothelium behaved as though it were 25 years older.

The moral (as many of my patients who have restored their energy and reduced their symptoms will tell you) is that you are never too young to be concerned about heart disease. And you are never too old to do something about it.

Your body holds the key to heart health. The Cardiovascular Cure is a healthy endothelium. This book will show you how to harness the power of nitric oxide and strengthen your endothelium, your body's self-defense against heart attack and stroke.

The Power of NO—
a Revolutionary
Breakthrough in
Cardiovascular
Medicine

Chapter 1

Your Blood Vessels and NO
(and Why You Need to Know about Them)

T HIS IS a story about the health of your blood vessels. If you are like most people, you have probably given some thought to the health of your heart, but not the 100,000 miles of blood vessels that run throughout your body. Wherever blood flows in your body, it flows through blood vessels.

Blood vessels have been given short shrift mainly because people think that they are nothing more than passive pipes. But we now know that they are much more important than anyone ever realized.

Your blood vessels are dynamic, living tissue just like any other organ in your body. And just like every other organ, they perform a vital function: in this case, controlling blood flow from one moment to the next. Every 60 seconds, your vessels are responsible for distributing five quarts of life-sustaining blood to your body. Just think, five quarts every minute, 1,800 gallons every day, a virtual river of life.

Composed of living cells, blood is alive. And like all living things, blood has its own complex functions. It carries the oxygen and nutrients your tissues need to survive. It removes the waste products of cellular metabolism, distributing these to the liver or kidney where the waste products can be excreted. Blood carries hormones from the brain and other glands to distant parts of the body where these hormones are needed for the growth and function of each organ. When you cut yourself, blood has the ability to clot and stop the bleeding. And when you lose blood, your body has the ability to make new blood, replacing what's been lost. Blood carries white blood cells, your body's major defense against infection. White blood cells course through all of the blood vessels, constantly patrolling for foreign invaders. If you think about it, blood is the unifying force within the body, both a link between distant parts and an intricate system of transportation that provides fuel, disposes of waste, and carries disease-fighting cells.

And all of this happens within the blood vessels.

As the conduit, blood vessels play a role in the ability of the blood to do its job. Blood vessels can control their own diameter and control the flow of blood from one moment to the next. They can open up to increase the flow of blood to where it is needed (such as to the muscles during exercise or to the pelvis during sexual intercourse). Blood vessels can also reduce the flow of blood to an area of the body. The blood vessels to the skin constrict or shut down completely when blood must be diverted (which is why a person may become pale with fear when blood is diverted from the skin to the muscles, heart, and brain where it is needed for fight or flight). Blood vessels can do this because their walls are made of muscle, similar to that of the heart muscle. This muscle responds to nervous impulses from the brain, to changes in pressure within the vessel, and to substances made by the endothelium, the inner lining of the blood vessels.

Blood vessels are always active and constantly in motion as they respond to the rhythms of the body: the heart, the flow of blood, signals from the brain, and signals from tissues of the body that need more blood. Like so many other parts of the body, blood vessels do their job without our conscious knowledge.

The small and large blood vessels perform different roles. The smaller vessels contract to restrict blood flow and dilate to increase it. They direct the flow of blood where it is needed. On the other hand, the larger vessels do not contract or dilate very much on their own, but instead respond to the beat of the heart. They expand with each beat, much as the inner tube of a tire expands when it is filled with air. When the heart relaxes between beats, the walls of the great vessels (the aorta, which carries blood from the heart to the rest of the body, and the pulmonary artery, which carries blood to the lungs) rebound, giving the blood an extra push forward, maintaining blood flow until the heart pumps again. (When you take your pulse, you are actually measuring the wave of energy that passes through the blood from the beating heart, expanding the vessels as the wave passes through.)

It is this dance between the heart and the great vessels that makes a smooth and efficient circulation system. To do their job properly—keeping pace with the heart, expanding and rebounding—vessels need to be pliable and elastic. You want your vessels to be as resilient as possible.

The problem is that—due to many factors, such as aging, genetics, poor diet, smoking, and sedentary lifestyle—the elasticity and flexibility of your vessels can become compromised. When vessels are the opposite of pliable and elastic, they are stiff and fixed in place like a pipe. When vessels are stiff, they can't comply with the beat of the heart and the waves of life-giving energy. When the heart pumps blood into stiff arteries, the heart must work harder. It takes more energy to pump blood through stiff vessels.

Although the smaller vessels do not harden like the larger ones, they can also become damaged and function poorly. Poor diet, lack of exercise, and risk factors such as aging, high blood pressure, high blood sugar, high cholesterol, and smoking all impair the ability of the smaller vessels to relax. The vessel wall becomes thicker and the bore of the vessels becomes smaller. The vessels tend to constrict rather than dilate, and it is more difficult for blood to flow through them. Accordingly, to get the same amount of blood flow through these vessels, the heart has to pump harder. As a result, blood pressure rises.

For hundreds of years, we've known that blood pressure is a measure of the blood circulating through the body. It is determined by the amount of blood flow and the blood vessels' resistance to that blood flow. The pumping of the heart establishes the amount of blood flow. When the heart beats faster or contracts more vigorously, blood flow increases. The health of the blood vessels determines the resistance. When the vessels are relaxed and flexible, resistance is low. In about 90 percent of people with high blood pressure, blood pressure increases because the vessels are not relaxed or have thickened.

You are probably familiar with the way blood pressure is measured. The measurement is represented by two numbers, top and bottom. The top number is the systolic pressure, the pressure in the vessels at the time the heart beats and pumps blood into the arteries. The bottom number, or diastolic pressure, is a measurement taken when the heart is resting in between beats. The normal blood pressure reading for an adult is 140/80; anything over these numbers is considered elevated.

In my opinion, the lower your blood pressure, the better. Obviously, if your blood pressure is too low, you will faint. But I tell my patients that their blood pressure should be just high enough to keep them from falling over. Even if your blood pressure is as low as 90/60 but you can stand without trouble, this is healthy and, in the long run, better for your heart and vessels.

To understand the difference between arteries that are stiff and those that are compliant, think about the difference between a thick and thin balloon. It is difficult to blow air into a thick-walled balloon. Expanding a thick-walled balloon takes much more effort than expanding a thin one, and the thick-walled balloon doesn't recoil very far once it is stretched. Like the thick-walled balloon, arteries that have hardened take much more effort to expand—and that makes it more difficult for the heart to pump blood into them. When blood is pumped into vessels that are not compliant, blood pressure rises faster and higher. The vessels can't expand to accommodate the rush of blood. On the other hand, the thin-walled balloon expands, stretches, and recoils with ease. It should be obvious then that, to maintain cardiovascular health, we want our vessels to be pliable like the thin-walled balloon. As you'll find out, it is possible to return your blood vessels to their youthful state.

The Lining of the Blood Vessel—the Endothelium

IF YOU were to look at the outside of a blood vessel, it would appear enmeshed and attached to surrounding tissue, almost as though it had a myriad of threads circling it. The inside of a blood vessel is different, made up of smooth tissue, the easier to facilitate the flow of blood.

A closer look inside a blood vessel takes us to the endothelium, the innermost layer of tissue that lines the blood vessel. If you were to look at a cross section of an artery, the endothelium would be the inner surface. It would be similar to looking into a garden hose: the inside of the hose is lined by a smooth surface that is like the endothelium.

All blood vessels are lined with a carpet of endothelial cells. The blood vessels in your skin, brain, heart, and all of your organs are lined with this film of tissue. Only one cell layer thick, the endothelium seems almost immaterial, so thin that it cannot be seen by the naked eye. Yet it is a fascinating, versatile, and vital part of our anatomy. It could even be considered the largest organ in our body. Because this almost invisible veil of tissue lines all blood vessels, and because we have about 100,000 miles of blood vessels, the endothelium has the surface area of eight tennis courts. Incredibly, if all of the endothelial cells in the body were lumped together, they would weigh as much as the liver.

For many years, researchers believed that the endothelium was nothing more than an inert layer of cells, a simple barrier between blood and the smooth muscle wall of the vessel. Nevertheless, the process through which this "barrier" worked fascinated physiologists for many years—ever since it was found that certain substances seemed to pass through it, whereas others could not. It acted as a selective filter for the vessel wall. Eventually, scientists suspected that the endothelium was more than just "wallpaper," as it had been called.

In 1966, Nobel laureate Lord Howard Walter Florey, honored in 1945 for discovering penicillin, predicted that we would eventually see "a rich harvest of new knowledge about the cells which stand between the blood and lymph streams and the cells of the tissue." No longer would endothelial cells be regarded as "little more than a sheet of nucleated cellophane," Florey wrote.[1]

Florey's words were prophetic. We now know that the endothelium exerts tremendous control over blood flow. First, its prime location plays a role. Because the endothelium is the innermost lining of the blood vessel, it has direct contact with blood and, as such, serves as an interface between the blood and the vessel wall. That relationship is everything, providing a clue to many details about the endothelium's job.

One detail in particular proved interesting to scientists studying the endothelium in the 1950s and was noted by Lord Florey in the 1960s: there was something special about endothelial cells since they permitted certain substances to pass through their barrier. Lord Florey even hinted in 1966 that "endothelial permeability may be of importance in elucidating the initial phases of the development of atherosclerosis."

But the endothelium is much more than a highly selective filter. We now know that this delicate tissue, only one cell layer in thickness, is a dynamic factory, producing a myriad of substances that maintain vessel health. It is, in essence, a silver lining—since when it's healthy, it produces its own forms of heart medicine.[2]

A Major Advance in Cardiovascular Medicine— the Discovery of NO/EDRF

THIS NEW chapter in cardiovascular medicine began with dynamite. In 1860, Alfred Nobel successfully made nitroglycerin explode. Six years later, he invented dynamite, using nitroglycerin as the active ingredient. Even then, in Alfred Nobel's time, scientists knew that small amounts of nitroglycerin could be given to relieve angina, but they didn't know how nitroglycerin worked. Somehow small doses of the explosive relaxed the muscles of the blood vessels, enabling the vessels to dilate. In people who had angina, nitroglycerin relieved the pain of the heart, which was starved of oxygen and nutrients.

Late in life, Alfred Nobel himself developed angina and took nitroglycerin for pain relief. "Isn't it the irony of fate that I have been prescribed nitroglycerin, to be taken internally," Nobel wrote to a colleague before he died of a heart attack in 1896. "They call it Trinitrin, so as not to scare the chemist and the public."[3]

But it wasn't until the 1970s that scientists began to uncover the mystery of how nitroglycerin worked. It was Dr. Ferid Murad, at the University of Virginia and later at Stanford University, who made the great leap forward in solving this medical puzzle.

Early on in Dr. Murad's career, he became interested in how cells signal to one another. "I decided to work with cyclic GMP [guanosine monophosphate] since it was emerging as a possible new second messenger to mediate hormone effects," he writes in *Les Prix Nobel,* a publication of the Nobel Foundation.[4]

"Second messengers" are molecules that are involved in carrying a message from the outside of the cell to the inside. For example, when adrenaline circulates in the blood, it binds to the outside surface of cells in the vessels and the heart. When it binds to the cell surface, it triggers the production of a second messenger just below the surface of the cell. The second messenger then spreads throughout the cell to pass on the message. Cyclic AMP (adenosine monophosphate) is the "second messenger" for adrenaline; it passes on the message of adrenaline to activate the fight-or-flight response.

In his work with cyclic GMP, Dr. Murad found that it was, in fact, the "second messenger" for NO. When NO enters a cell, it activates an enzyme called guanylate cyclase, which produces the second messenger, cyclic GMP. In this way, cyclic GMP does the work of NO; it relaxes muscle cells. In effect, Dr. Murad had solved the mystery of how nitroglycerin causes blood vessels to relax. He had found that nitroglycerin released NO, which increased the activity of an enzyme (guanylate cyclase) that caused a chain reaction, resulting in relaxed muscle tissue.

This was a startling new finding because up until that time NO was mainly thought of as a product of car exhaust, a toxic gas that existed only outside the body. It was considered a poison and, to some, a nuisance. (Years later, Dr. Murad's discovery would have an impact on a new drug called Viagra. Viagra improves erections by increasing blood flow to the penis; it does this by preventing the breakdown of cyclic GMP. By extending the action of cyclic GMP, Viagra assists the action of nitric oxide, thus improving blood flow to the penis.)

At about the time that Dr. Murad was putting finishing touches on his work, another researcher, Dr. Robert Furchgott, a pharmacologist at the State University of New York (SUNY) in Brooklyn, and his assistant made a surprising observation. In the laboratory they were studying the contraction of blood vessels using animal models. Blood vessels are harvested and studied in special chambers filled with aerated salt solution to keep them alive and functioning. They are hooked up to sensitive transducers to measure their contraction. For most of the experiments, Dr. Furchgott and his assistant prepared the vessels in the traditional way, cutting them into helical strips. Then, during the studies, they observed the vessels contracting. But one fateful day, they skipped this step and instead simply cut the vessels into small sections. When they did the experiment, the vessels relaxed instead of contracted. Dr. Furchgott puzzled over this strange result and, in subsequent days, repeated it. They eventually realized that, unknowingly, they had kept the endothelium intact when they cut the vessels into small sections and not helical strips. Dr. Furchgott realized that the presence of the endothelium made all the difference in how the vessels behaved. They found that the endothelium was making a powerful vessel relaxant that "signaled" smooth muscles in the arteries and told them to relax. Dr. Furchgott called this substance "endothelium-derived relaxing factor," or EDRF.[5]

When his work was published in 1980, it set off a race in laboratories around the world to discover the identity of EDRF. It would take six years for scientists to figure it out. One of the reasons that EDRF remained a mystery was that it was extremely short-lived, persisting for only fractions of a second in the vessel wall. So Dr. Furchgott could not initially identify what EDRF was.

During those six years, scientists came ever closer to realizing similarities between EDRF and nitric oxide. The ultimate experiments to prove that they were one and the same were performed independently by Dr. Furchgott and Dr. Louis Ignarro at the University of California at Los Angeles. In 1986, both men provided evidence that EDRF and NO were the same molecule. EDRF and NO had similar characteristics: they both caused blood vessel dilation, they were both short-lived and decayed in a matter of seconds, and they both reacted in the same way to a host of other chemicals.

(NO/EDRF was not the first vasodilator that had been discovered within the endothelium. In 1976, a research group led by Sir John Vane published its observation that the vessel wall could make its own vasodilator. Sir John went on to isolate and characterize the substance as prostacyclin, derived from the metabolism of arachidonic acid [a fatty acid]. For this seminal work, Sir John and two other scientists received the Nobel Prize in 1982. Prostacyclin, a sister molecule of EDRF, is another weapon in the endothelium's arsenal against vascular disease.)

The discovery of NO/EDRF was an extremely important one—it was the first time that a gas had been found to act as a signaling molecule in the body, easily crossing between cell membranes. In addition, NO/EDRF played a critical role in cardiovascular function. On October 12, 1998, three Americans—Furchgott, Ignarro, and Murad—were awarded the Nobel Prize for the discovery that nitric oxide could act as a signal to many cells in the body. The Nobel Committee at the Karolinska Institute in Stockholm said that the discovery of these three scientists had "elicited an avalanche of research activities in many different laboratories around the world." They also explained that the research had led to new treatments in heart and lung diseases, shock, and impotence.[6]

The three Americans were hailed for their discoveries concerning "nitric oxide as a signalling molecule in the cardiovascular system." With the work of these scientists, the field of cardiovascular medicine took a great leap forward. "The discovery of nitric oxide and its function is one of the most important in the history of cardiovascular medicine," Dr. Valentin Fuster, then president of the American

Heart Association, told the *New York Times*.[7] And most everyone in the field of cardiovascular medicine agreed.

What NO/EDRF Can Do for You (and Your Blood Vessels)

THE WORK of the Nobel Prize–winning scientists had revealed that a healthy endothelium releases its own form of nitroglycerin. Heart patients are familiar with nitroglycerin. When they have an angina attack, they slip a tablet of nitroglycerin under their tongue, where it rapidly dissolves and enters their blood system. A person with heart disease can get almost immediate relief from chest pain because the nitroglycerin releases NO into the vessels to relax them. The heart vessels relax and deliver more blood flow to the heart muscle.

NO is the body's own form of nitroglycerin. In fact, heart patients would not need to take nitroglycerin if their vessels were making enough NO. I sometimes tell heart patients to think of a healthy endothelium as a lifelong supply of nitroglycerin. But having a healthy endothelium is much better than taking nitroglycerin. Nature takes much better care of blood vessels than do drugs.

When blood vessels produce NO by themselves, they release NO in response to the rhythms of the body. Small amounts of NO are released directly where it is needed. The production of NO by the vessel wall is tightly controlled by nerve stimulation, circulating hormones, and the tissue that the vessel serves.

By contrast, taking the medicine known as nitroglycerin is like exposing all of your vessels at once to a shotgun blast of NO. A nitroglycerin pill is effective in relieving chest pain in someone who has heart disease. But if it relaxes the blood vessel too much, it can lower blood pressure so much that the patient faints. Furthermore, prolonged and daily use of drugs similar to nitroglycerin can damage the ability of your vessels to produce their own supply of NO.

I do give some of my heart patients a short-acting form of nitroglycerin to put under their tongue during an attack. But I also encourage them to improve their endothelial health so that they can make their own NO. In addition, I generally avoid prescribing long-acting nitrates, because when these are taken on a daily basis for a prolonged period of time, they can impair the body's own supply of NO.

NO/EDRF's Contribution to Cardiovascular Health

THE NOBEL laureates won their prize for discovering that NO is a potent relaxer of blood vessels. But since this landmark finding, we have learned much more about how NO contributes to cardiovascular health. We have also learned how to improve the production of this lifesaving molecule through nutrition and lifestyle changes.

Based on the work of many research groups, including my own, we now know that when someone has heart disease or risk factors for heart disease, their endothelium is impaired. When the endothelium is not healthy, the vessel constricts and, over time, the vessel wall thickens. Blood cells are more likely to stick to the vessel, and this accumulation may lead to the formation of a blood clot or the development of atherosclerotic plaque.

However, when the endothelium is healthy, it releases NO, which relaxes the blood vessels, prevents cells from sticking to the vessel wall, and prevents the vessel wall from thickening.

A healthy endothelium is like Teflon, a nonstick surface that enhances the flow of blood. By contrast, an unhealthy endothelium is like Velcro, with white blood cells and platelets sticking to it. Together, NO and its sister molecule prostacyclin act together to maintain the vessel in a relaxed state and to prevent the development of blood clots and plaque.

What exactly does NO do for your blood vessels?

NO opens blood vessels and keeps them relaxed. To keep your circulatory system as healthy as possible, you will want your blood vessels to be as relaxed and pliable as possible. NO is the strongest natural relaxant of blood vessels. By causing blood vessels to open up, NO increases blood flow through them. As a cardiologist I have several vasodilating drugs that I can administer to my patients. I use these drugs to improve blood flow and to lower blood pressure. But by ensuring that your body makes NO on its own, you have a natural vasodilator right in your own body. Like nitroglycerin, NO acts on the blood vessels immediately.

NO prevents atherosclerosis. NO is a natural substance that protects us from hardening of the arteries. It does this by preventing platelets (particles in the blood that form blood clots) and white blood cells from sticking to the vessel wall. NO also reduces the production of free radicals, which can cause your vessels to age rapidly.

NO also suppresses the abnormal growth of vascular muscle cells, which can thicken the vessel. All of these processes—the sticking of blood cells to the vessel, the production of free radicals, and abnormal cell growth—contribute to atherosclerosis. (For more information on what causes atherosclerosis, see Chapter 3.) By halting these processes, endothelium-made NO is your body's strongest self-defense against heart attack and stroke. NO can prevent hardening of the arteries and even reverse it. This process may take some time and is one of the long-term benefits of NO.

THE LAST few years have been exciting for me and for other scientists working in this area of vascular medicine. We have uncovered many secrets of the body and the blood vessels. However, it is even more gratifying for me to use these secrets to enhance vessel health. I believe that it is important for people to learn how to enhance the healing power within—and to benefit from the body's natural defense against heart attack and stroke. It is for this reason that I created the program for endothelial health, an evidence-based, scientifically designed diet, exercise, and nutritional supplement program. Based on the research of the Nobel laureates, my laboratory, and many others, the endothelial health program is designed to stimulate the natural mechanism within our bodies that can fight vascular disease of all kinds, including peripheral artery disease, coronary artery disease, and stroke.

Can NO help you? The answer is yes—by helping to keep your vessels relaxed and open and by preventing atherosclerosis. It is never too late to learn about the power of NO. I have seen people with very unhealthy blood vessels become more healthy. The endothelium can be repaired. Atherosclerosis can be reversed.

When the lining of the blood vessels in healthy cells don't stick, clots don't form, arteries don't harden, and you won't die of a heart attack or stroke. The cardiovascular cure is a healthy endothelium. This is certainly promising news for all of us.

VIEW FROM THE RED BLOOD CELL
(AND HOW IT CIRCULATES)

To help you visualize how the circulation system works, let's take a ride on a red blood cell.

A red blood cell is exceedingly small. Seven million of these disc-shaped cells can easily fit into a thimble. Our little lifeboat is bright red because it is filled with oxygen. We begin in the left ventricle. As the ventricles contract, we are forcibly expelled through the aortic valve and out into the aorta, where we are swept along with billions of other red blood cells.

The force of this rushing blood (the heart pumps approximately one cup of blood with each heartbeat) expands the elastic wall of the aorta in much the same manner as an inner tube of a tire expands with air. Behind us, the left ventricle has finished its contraction and begins to relax. The aortic valve closes, and for a fraction of a second we pause in our headlong flight through the aorta. But as the elastic wall of the aorta rebounds, the current picks up speed again and we rush forward.

As we stream along in this bright red river, we pass many branches of the aorta. The first two branches are the left and right coronary arteries, which supply the heart muscle with blood. Then we pass the branch that supplies blood to the right arm and right carotid artery. (The carotid arteries supply the head with blood.)

As we course over the arch of the aorta, we pass the left carotid (which supplies blood to the brain) and the branch that supplies blood to the left arm. Now we move down the aorta toward the chest, abdomen, and legs. Along the way we pass branches that supply the spine, gut, and pelvis with blood. Up ahead, there is a fork in the road as the aorta bifurcates into the two arteries that supply the pelvis and legs with blood. This time we exit into the main artery of the right leg.

Moving down this artery, we pass many branches and find ourselves in the right foot. Our tributary now is about one-sixth of an inch in diameter, in comparison with the aorta, which was two inches in diameter at the left ventricle (and about one inch before it divided into the two branches to the legs).

Our artery branches again and again as we travel deeper into the right foot. At last, we find ourselves in a threadlike vessel (an arteriole) that is supplying the skin of the right big toe. This thread-like vessel branches again and again until we find ourselves in a vessel not visible to the naked eye, a capillary. The capillary vessel wall is only one cell layer in thickness. Its diameter is so small (about 7 microns) that we can barely squeeze through.

Guess what this tiny vessel is made of? That's right, it's a tube of endothelial cell and is only one cell layer in thickness. The thinness of the capillary permits nutrients to quickly pass from the blood into the tissue.

As our red blood cell passes through this capillary, it begins to give up its oxygen. Fluids and nutrients in the plasma that surround our red blood cell also leak through the capillary walls. In this way, the surrounding tissue receives the oxygen and nutrients it needs to survive. As the capillary winds its way through the tissue, carbon dioxide and other waste products from the tissue diffuse through the capillary walls and into the bloodstream.

The velocity of our transit has slowed considerably from about three feet per second (in the aorta) to one inch per second (in the capillaries). The slower flow in the capillaries provides ample time for the exchange of nutrients from the blood to the tissue. We darken as we give up oxygen. We have now squeezed through the capillary, and the vessel through which we are flowing begins to get larger as it joins other small vessels. We are now traveling in a venule (small vein) before making our way back toward the heart.

The venules join to form veins. The vein we are in crosses the top surface of the foot, curves around the ankle, and rises up the inner calf and thigh. These veins are directing the blood back to the heart. Many of the larger veins have one-way valves to ensure that the blood goes forward to the heart rather than pooling in the legs. When these valves leak, blood tends to pool in the leg and distends the veins. Over time, the veins can become enlarged (varicose veins are usually caused by leaky valves).

The veins traverse the pelvis and merge to form the inferior vena cava. This large vein (one to one and a half inches in diameter) accepts tributaries from the abdomen and thorax before it empties into the right side of the heart, into the right atrium (the collecting chamber adjacent to the right ventricle). When the right ventricle relaxes, a valve opens and the red blood cells stream from the right atrium into the right ventricle. Next, the right ventricle begins to contract, forcing open the pulmonary valve. We are ejected into the pulmonary (lung) artery and its branches.

As we travel deeper into the lung, the branches we take become smaller and once again we find ourselves in vessels the size of threads. We flow along past even more forks in the stream and eventually find ourselves once again squeezing through capillaries. However, now the surrounding tissue (the lung) is filled with oxygen, which diffuses into our red blood cell and turns it bright red again. We expel carbon dioxide (a waste product picked up in the body's tissues) into the lung.

We then flow out of the lung capillaries through venules that grow larger in diameter as they join other tributaries—all on their way back to the heart. Now we are in the pulmonary veins that direct oxygenated blood into the left atrium (the collecting chamber adjacent to the left ventricle). When the left ventricle relaxes, a valve opens and we stream into this thick-walled cavity. Now the left ventricle contracts forcefully and we are ejected through the aortic valve—to begin our journey through the body again.

Chapter 2

The Scientific Basis
for the Nutritional Program

ALTHOUGH THE Nobel Prize was awarded in 1998 for the discovery of NO, the history of this molecule, and the discoveries surrounding it, extend back 20 years—ever since the late 1970s, when Dr. Furchgott first discovered that the endothelium made a powerful vessel relaxant. What follows is the story of how my laboratory, and others around the world, built on Dr. Furchgott's discovery and devised new treatments for endothelial health.

The Other Important Discovery—
the Case for L-Arginine

WE KNEW what the endothelium was supposed to do. But sometimes it didn't work properly. Sometimes it didn't relax the blood vessel. Scientists were determined to find out why. Throughout the mid-1980s, there was a flurry of research to find out what could interfere with the normal functioning of the endothelium.

In 1988, I was an assistant professor of medicine at Harvard; I had my own small laboratory and was just getting started as an independent investigator. Research teams from around the world were working to figure out what caused the endothelium to become unhealthy. One team in Belgium found that the endothelium did not relax the vessel well, or function properly, in animals with high cholesterol. Another team at Harvard found that the endothelium didn't function well in patients with diseased coronary arteries. Expanding on the work of these researchers, my team found that, even in otherwise healthy young people, an increase in cholesterol level impaired the ability of the endothelium to relax the blood vessel.

These findings raised even more questions. How did high cholesterol harm the endothelium? And what, if anything, could we do about it?

In the spring of 1988, I traveled to Copper Mountain in Colorado for a scientific meeting that would answer some of these questions— and add a whole new dimension to our research. The surprise came during the presentation of Dr. Salvador Moncada of England, who announced that he had discovered the substance from which endothelium-derived nitric oxide is formed. The substance was an amino acid, known as L-arginine, that can be found in protein.[1]

L-arginine is a semi-essential amino acid. Our bodies are capable of making some of the L-arginine we need, but we also need additional L-arginine from the protein foods we eat. (Unfortunately, most Americans obtain their L-arginine largely from red meat. As you will learn in later chapters, there are more healthful sources of this important amino acid. See Chapter 4 for more information on foods containing L-arginine.)

L-Arginine Makes NO and Improves Blood Vessel Dilation

I WAS excited by Dr. Moncada's presentation at the Copper Mountain meeting. If he was right and L-arginine could convert to NO in the body, what would happen if we gave L-arginine to people with high cholesterol? Could we boost the production of NO? If the answer was yes, we would have a simple way of improving blood vessel health.

I wanted to put these questions to the test immediately. During the coffee break following Dr. Moncada's presentation, I called Boston and asked my lab assistant to order a supply of L-arginine.

After successfully testing the hypothesis in animals, we performed an experiment to find out whether L-arginine could improve the dilation of blood vessels in people with high cholesterol. We divided people into two groups, giving one an intravenous solution of salt water and the other an intravenous infusion of salt water and

L-arginine. To stimulate the endothelium to produce nitric oxide, we used a chemical called acetylcholine, infused into the artery. We then measured the increase in blood flow to the arm with a strain gauge apparatus, a mercury-filled tube placed around the forearm that can detect blood flow.

In the people given salt water, the ability of their blood vessels to relax (already poor from high cholesterol) was not improved by the infusion. (Saline, the liquid used to deliver L-arginine, has no effect of its own on vascular reaction.) However, to our great satisfaction, in the people receiving L-arginine, blood flow was restored to normal within minutes of the infusion (even though it had no effect on cholesterol level). The speed at which this happened, and the level of improvement in these patients' endothelial function, created a lot of excitement in the lab. We were beginning to realize the power of L-arginine; even in patients whose blood vessels were impaired by high cholesterol, L-arginine increased production of nitric oxide, which improved vessel health. It was remarkable that an amino acid could help restore blood flow at all, let alone so rapidly.

THE ARGININE PARADOX (WHO NEEDS L-ARGININE?)

While we were engaged in these studies with L-arginine, Dr. Ulrich Forstermann, a German scientist then at the Abbott Laboratories in Illinois, performed a series of experiments isolating nitric oxide synthase (NOS), the enzyme that makes nitric oxide. He found that only small amounts of L-arginine are necessary to make NO (the NOS enzyme reached half of its full activity when L-arginine was present at concentrations that were only 5 percent of what is seen in our blood). His studies suggested that there was plenty of L-arginine in our blood to make NO.

We found that this was true in people with healthy vessels. In these individuals, L-arginine did not further improve vasodilation. But what about people at risk for, or who had, heart disease? In these people, we found that additional L-arginine did improve blood flow. Apparently, the amount of L-arginine circulating in their blood was insufficient. The discrepancy between Forstermann's work and ours became known as the arginine paradox: there is enough L-arginine present in the blood to make NO, but people with unhealthy vessels make more NO when given L-arginine. The paradox was resolved a few years later with the discovery of

ADMA, a molecule circulating in the blood of people with, or at risk of, heart disease (see p. 23). ADMA opposes the action of L-arginine. In the meantime, we began to learn more about how L-arginine could improve people's lives.

The First Evidence That
L-Arginine Improves Symptoms

WHEN I spoke about our experiments with L-arginine at scientific meetings in 1989, I was met with skepticism. However, over the next few years, other investigators tested our hypothesis and came up with the same results in people with high cholesterol or people with disease of the heart and limb vessels. In the early 1990s, it became clear to the scientific community that giving patients L-arginine could improve blood flow and vessel relaxation in certain types of patients.

Once we had performed the initial studies showing that supplemental L-arginine could improve blood flow in people with high cholesterol, we were eager to see if it could improve patients' symptoms. Among the first research groups to show the benefit of L-arginine in people's lives were Drs. Rainer Boger and Stephanie Bode-Boger at the University of Hannover in 1996. They found that, in patients with peripheral arterial disease, intravenous L-arginine increased blood flow to the legs. The benefit of giving L-arginine was equivalent to that of giving the drug prostaglandin E1 (widely used in Europe to treat poor blood flow to the legs). In a second study, they found that L-arginine was at least as effective as the drug at improving the ability of these patients to walk.

Still another research team, this one at the Mayo Clinic, found that patients with angina who were given L-arginine had a 150 percent increase in coronary blood flow response to acetylcholine and a 60 percent reduction in the frequency of angina symptoms. And, on top of that, their symptoms improved within one week of taking L-arginine supplements.

In parallel, at Stanford, we were finding that L-arginine supplementation could reduce the stickiness of platelets and white blood cells in people with high cholesterol.

The news about L-arginine was promising.[2] These studies suggested that there was a new way to improve blood flow, reduce symptoms of heart disease, and enhance endothelial health.

The Long-Term Benefits of Nitric Oxide— Reversing Heart Disease

IN 1990, when I first got to Stanford, I began to work on the long-term effects of enhancing NO production. We had evidence of many of the short-term benefits, but could there be other, long-term benefits to enhancing NO?

I thought that if we could improve NO synthesis over a long period of time, we could slow hardening of the arteries. We set to work and, within a year, were able to confirm this hypothesis.

NO slows plaque growth and suppresses atherosclerosis. In experiments using animals with high cholesterol, we found that those given L-arginine developed markedly less plaque than those that were given placebo. Intriguingly, L-arginine did not change the amount of cholesterol in the blood, which showed that cholesterol is not the sole determinant of whether or not atherosclerosis develops.

Other experiments provided us with insight into the molecular mechanism through which vascular NO could suppress atherosclerosis. We found that the blood vessels of animals fed a high-fat diet had a stickier lining than vessels of animals fed a healthy diet. Specifically, we observed that the white blood cells of animals with high cholesterol were more likely to cling to the vessel lining. However, the white blood cells were less likely to stick when L-arginine was added to the high-fat diet. Vessels treated with L-arginine made less cellular Velcro. In the L-arginine-treated animals, the Teflon-like quality of the vessel lining was restored.

By reducing the stickiness of the endothelium, NO prevents white blood cells and platelets from clinging to the vessel wall. This is important because it is the invasion of the white blood cells into the vessel wall, and their battle with cholesterol, that leads to plaque formation. It is the stickiness of the platelets, which form blood clots, that contributes to heart attack and stroke.

In essence, NO calms the cells flowing through the vessel and, in so doing, protects the vessel wall. Even when blood cholesterol is high, if the vessel is producing sufficient amounts of NO, the vessel will be protected from the development of plaque. These studies suggest that if we can maintain the health of the endothelium, and the production of NO, we are protected from atherosclerosis even in the face of high levels of cholesterol.

When in 1992 we reported the results about L-arginine slowing plaque growth, the scientific community was appropriately skeptical. Any new finding needs to be confirmed or disproved by other scientists. Only after a new finding has been tested by other scientists is it accepted by the scientific community. One very good scientist, who set out to prove us wrong, repeated our experiment. To his surprise, he got results that were identical to ours.

Since 1992, our studies showing that L-arginine slows plaque growth have been confirmed multiple times by laboratories around the world. These studies suggested that if we maintain the health of the endothelium, and the production of NO, we are protected from coronary disease.

NO melts away or shrinks plaque that is already there. Using animal models, we also found that L-arginine could get rid of, or shrink, plaque that had already built up in the vessels. *L-arginine actually had the ability to melt away plaque.* This occurred when L-arginine was taken up in the vessels that had been damaged by plaque. The cells in the damaged vessel were able to use the L-arginine to produce more NO. This increase in NO production not only prevented more white cells from coming in, it also caused the white blood cells in the vessel wall to die and fade away—it was this dying and fading away that melted the plaque. This was also a striking discovery, suggesting that increasing vascular NO production could prevent atherosclerosis and reverse the disease in people who already had it.

With the knowledge that a healthy endothelium protects us from atherosclerosis, we are armed with a new way to inhibit, slow, or even reverse the progression of atherosclerosis. A healthy endothelium is, in essence, the cardiovascular cure.

WHAT NO DOES FOR BLOOD VESSELS

In a healthy endothelium, NO does the following:

Keeps vessels pliable and elastic
Keeps blood flowing smoothly
Keeps platelets calm and prevents them from sticking to the vessel wall
Keeps white blood cells calm and prevents them from sticking to the vessel wall
Regulates oxidative enzymes in the cell, preventing oxidation
Reduces growth and multiplication of muscle cells that thicken the vessel wall
Slows plaque growth and suppresses atherosclerosis
May melt away plaque that already exists

A Series of Findings That Helped Me to Create the Nutritional Program

1. When NO Doesn't Go

What was the difference between people who were healthy and made enough NO on their own and people who were unhealthy and not producing enough NO? In 1992, Drs. Salvador Moncada and Patrick Vallance helped solve this puzzle when they discovered another amino acid that plays a big role in vascular disease. They found that the modified amino acid ADMA (asymmetric dimethylarginine) could block the production of NO.

For years, biochemists had known that ADMA was present in urine. Drs. Moncada and Vallance were the first to realize the significance of this observation. They found that patients with kidney failure, who are known to have accelerated hardening of the arteries and high risk for heart attack and stroke, cannot excrete ADMA and so have very high blood levels of it. Drs. Moncada and Vallance reasoned that this arginine-like molecule might block the effect of L-arginine. They were right.

In its composition, ADMA is identical to L-arginine, except that it has two extra methyl groups attached to it. Both ADMA and

L-arginine can attach to the enzyme NO synthase (NOS). When L-arginine attaches, it is converted to NO. When ADMA attaches, it cannot be converted to NO. It is a wrench in the machinery. It blocks the enzyme.

Conclusion: ADMA turns off the production of NO.

2. Who Has High ADMA Levels

After the observation by Drs. Moncada and Vallance that ADMA was elevated in people with kidney failure, the focus of research teams around the world, including ours, was to find out if ADMA was responsible for the lack of NO in people at risk for, or who had, heart disease.

Drs. Rainer Boger and Stephanie Bode-Boger at the University of Hannover in Germany found that ADMA levels were elevated in people with peripheral arterial disease. They found that the higher the blood level of ADMA, the worse the vessel disease. A short time later, Dr. Imaizumi and coworkers in Japan found the same to be true of brain arteries. Using ultrasound to observe blood vessels in the neck of 120 Japanese patients, Dr. Imaizumi found that the higher the blood level of ADMA, the thicker the plaque in the neck arteries. Recent work by Dr. Azuma's group in Tokyo revealed that blood ADMA level is an independent marker for vessel thickening in women.

We also collaborated with many different researchers from around the world and found that blood levels of ADMA were elevated in people with each of the risk factors for heart disease: high cholesterol, high triglycerides, high blood pressure, high blood sugar, insulin resistance, high homocysteine, and tobacco use.

Highlights of our findings include:

ADMA and high cholesterol. What was most interesting was the high correlation between the level of ADMA and the level of endothelial dsyfunction. We found that *the blood level of ADMA is a better predictor of endothelial impairment than the level of cholesterol*.

In a recent study with Drs. Mary and Marguerite Engler of the University of California at San Francisco (UCSF), we found that even young children with high cholesterol had endothelial dysfunction, a reminder that vascular problems start in childhood. Studies are underway to determine if these children also have high ADMA levels.

ADMA and triglycerides. Triglyceride is a common form of fat found in fatty foods and in the bloodstream. In a collaborative study with Dr. Pia Lundman and coworkers at the Karolinska Institute in Stockholm, we found that triglyceride levels are highly correlated with ADMA levels in the blood. In parallel, Dr. Ali Fard at Columbia University discovered that ADMA increases in the blood after eating a high-fat or high-carbohydrate meal. The level of fat in the blood peaks about two hours after the meal and remains elevated for about four to six hours. As a result, the endothelium functions poorly, which may be why so many heart disease patients complain of chest pain after eating a heavy meal, particularly if they have to perform some physical activity after the meal.

ADMA, blood sugar, and insulin. Working with Dr. Gerald Reaven of Stanford, we found that ADMA levels were high when there was insulin resistance. The level of ADMA correlates better with insulin resistance than with any other marker.

ADMA and homocysteine. With Dr. Rene Malinow and his group at Oregon Health Sciences, we found that ADMA levels correlate with homocysteine levels. We have since shown that homocysteine causes impairment of the endothelium by increasing ADMA levels. We measured endothelial function in patients with vascular disease before and after taking a dose of methionine (which converts to homocysteine in the body). After ingesting the methionine, homocysteine levels rose, ADMA went up, and endothelial function declined in vascular patients. We went on to find that homocysteine was directly responsible for the increase in ADMA. However, we found that the healthy subjects were resistant to methionine; their ADMA levels did not increase, nor did their endothelial function deteriorate. We concluded that if your endothelium is healthy, you could have a built-in resistance to things that impair endothelial health (such as an occasional large, high-fat meal).

ADMA and tobacco. We collaborated with Dr. Imaizumi's group in Japan and found that smokers have higher blood ADMA levels.

Conclusion: People with risk factors for heart disease or people with heart disease have high ADMA levels. In fact, we believe that ADMA is a common pathway through which all risk factors exert their adverse effect on the vessel wall. ADMA accumulates in people with risk factors. ADMA blocks the production of NO, causing poor blood flow and contributing to hardening of the arteries.

3. How the Body Deals with ADMA (and the Link to Oxidative Stress)
The body has two ways of getting rid of ADMA. It can be excreted in urine. And it can be broken down by the enzyme DDAH (dimethyl-arginine dimethylaminohydrolase). At Stanford, we have found that production of ADMA is balanced by the breakdown action of DDAH. If DDAH becomes reduced or impaired, ADMA gradually increases and constricts blood flow.

We found that all of the major risk factors for heart disease such as high blood levels of cholesterol, homocysteine, and blood sugar reduce the ability of DDAH to break down ADMA. This is because these risk factors cause oxidative stress. As it turns out, DDAH is exquisitely sensitive to oxidative stress—and its activity is reduced by it. We can restore DDAH activity by reducing oxidative stress.

Conclusion: If there is oxidative stress, ADMA accumulates. DDAH can be strengthened with antioxidants.

Multiple Causes of Poor Endothelial Health— Problems and Solutions

ADMA IS one way in which the endothelium can become dysfunctional. But there are other ways things that can go wrong; the degree and the type of dysfunction depends on age, sex, genetic makeup, and number of risk factors to which an individual has been exposed. Regardless of the type of injury, the endothelium can be restored. My endothelial health program incorporates all of the healthful strategies necessary to heal the endothelium and counteracts each of the things that can go wrong.

> **You may have**: Reduced production of NO due to ADMA.
> **You may need**: Antioxidants and L-arginine.
> **Why**: We know that oxidative stress weakens DDAH (the enzyme that helps the body get rid of ADMA). We also know that DDAH activity can be protected or enhanced by antioxidants (such as those in fruits and vegetables), improving the body's ability to get rid of ADMA. We also know that L-arginine can help reverse the problem of accumulated ADMA.

> **You may have**: Damage to the endothelium and destruction of NO by oxygen-derived free radicals.

You may need: Antioxidants (in particular flavonoids and carotenoids and other phytochemicals).

Why: High blood levels of cholesterol, triglyceride, sugar, and homocysteine activate enzymes in the endothelium to make free radicals. Some people are also genetically prone to make more free radicals. One of these free radicals, superoxide anion, combines with NO to convert it into a dangerous free radical, peroxynitrite anion (or OONO-). It is now clear that too much superoxide anion is produced in many of the conditions known to be risk factors for heart attack and stroke. This can be countered with antioxidants. As you will learn in later chapters, the best complex of antioxidants is obtained through a plant-based diet.

You may have: Reduced amounts of NO synthase enzyme in the vessel wall.

You may need: Exercise; phytoestrogens.

Why: In the vessels of people with advanced atherosclerosis or advanced pulmonary hypertension, there is markedly less NO synthase (the enzyme that makes NO). NO synthase can be thought of as the factory in your blood vessels that produces NO. In people with low levels of the enzyme NO synthase, L-arginine will not have any impact since the factory for turning L-arginine to NO is not operating. Exercise is the best way to naturally increase the amount of NO synthase in your vessel wall. There is evidence that phytoestrogens (from soy protein or soy supplements) can also enhance the NO synthase pathway.

You may have: Inadequate amounts of the cofactors for NO production.

You may need: B vitamins.

Why: Low levels of a substance called tetrahydrobiopterin (also known as BH4) can reduce the activity of NO synthase. We can restore BH4 levels with B vitamins, in particular folate. The B vitamins also are beneficial because they reduce the blood level of homocysteine, which is known to impair endothelial function. Homocysteine causes the production of free radicals, which destroy NO. Homocysteine also interferes with the body's ability to rid itself of ADMA.

You may have: Impaired vessel response to NO.

You may need: Soy, especially the phytoestrogens daidzein and genistein.

Why: As blood vessels become more diseased, their ability to respond to NO also becomes impaired. Even if NO is delivered directly to the vessel (such as with certain drugs like nitroglycerin), the ability of the vessel to relax in response to NO is poor. At Stanford, we have found that phytoestrogens (especially daidzein and genistein) in soy protein can markedly improve the ability of the vessel to respond to NO.

You may have: Inadequate production of other endothelial protective factors.
You may need: Omega-3 fatty acids and an exercise program.
Why: There are other substances besides NO that can help protect the vessel. One of these is prostacyclin (PGI_2), which is similar to NO in that it relaxes blood vessels, increases blood flow, and prevents platelets from clumping in the vessels and white blood cells from sticking. It also prevents abnormal multiplication of the vascular cells, thereby preventing thickening of the vessel. You can help your body make more prostacyclin by ensuring that you get enough omega-3 fatty acids in your diet. Another protective factor is superoxide dismutase (SOD). SOD, which helps the body dispose of free radicals, can be increased through a proper exercise program.

You may have: Overproduction by the body of substances that cause vessels to spasm and/or to thicken.
You may need: Omega-3 fatty acids, L-arginine, and phytochemical antioxidants.
Why: When the endothelium is unhealthy, it makes fewer protective factors and more substances that cause the vessels to spasm. If the endothelium is unhealthy for a long time, these vasospastic factors will also accelerate thickening of the vessel. Many of the substances that have a rapid effect on vessel motion also have long-term effects on vessel structure. Substances such as NO and prostacyclin, which relax the vessel, also prevent thickening. Substances such as endothelin (ET, a protein produced by the endothelium) and thromboxane (TX, a lipid peroxide produced by the endothelium) cause vessels to spasm, and in the long term, they also cause vessels to thicken. A healthy vessel makes NO and PGI_2 and is relaxed and pliable. A sick vessel makes TX and ET and is constricted and thickened. My program for endothelial health tips the balance in favor of NO and PGI_2.

The program that I have designed for endothelial health takes advantage of what we have learned over the past 20 years about the endothelium. It is a natural way to restore vessel health in people, young or old, healthy or ill. If you are healthy, the program will maintain and enhance your health and protect you from vascular disease. If you are at risk for vascular disease, it will restore the health of your vessels. And if you already have vascular disease, or have already had a heart attack or stroke, this program will help repair your blood vessels, prevent another heart attack or stroke, and enhance the heart medicines that your doctor recommends.

Chapter 3

Facing the Enemy, Atherosclerosis

M R. JIM Y., 38, was scared. He sat in my office, worried and upset, and told me about his symptoms. The burning chest discomfort, which had started four days ago following exertion or stress, would ease up when he sat down and relaxed. With the least bit of physical activity, he experienced shortness of breath. After climbing just one flight of stairs, he found himself gasping. "When my wife saw that, she sent me here," he said, smiling sheepishly.

This was not Jim's first visit to a cardiologist. Two years earlier, he had gone to the emergency room with similar symptoms. In the ER, he was given nitroglycerin and morphine to relieve the pain. Blood studies and an EKG revealed that he had suffered a small heart attack. He was hospitalized for a few days and given intravenous medicine to lower his heart rate and blood pressure. He went home with instructions to take an aspirin daily and a beta-blocker, a common drug prescribed to lower heart rate and blood pressure.

After this scare, Jim stopped smoking. Since then, he felt reasonably well and returned to his work as a semiconductor technician. He liked his job, but it was largely sedentary. He admitted that he was not very careful about what he ate.

As I examined him, I noted that Jim, an Asian who weighed 203 pounds and measured 5 feet 10 inches, was overweight. (Based on his height and weight, Jim had a body mass index [BMI] of 29 kg/m^2, which put him in the overweight range. Overweight begins at a BMI of 25 kg/m². See Chapter 4 for more information on body mass index.)

Nevertheless, his blood pressure—112/76—was good. Given his level of stress and lack of exercise, I had expected his resting heart rate to be faster than 68 beats per minute. His low heart rate and blood pressure were probably due to the beta-blocker. Despite his history of smoking for 10 years, his lungs were clear and his heart sounds were normal.

When I asked Jim about his family's health, he said that his wife and two young daughters were in good health. But then he looked me squarely in the eye and told me his father had succumbed to a heart attack at age 69, his mother at age 55, and all of his uncles in their 50s. His older brother had had open heart bypass surgery when he was 38. There was no doubt that Jim had a strong and disturbing family history of heart disease.

I told Jim that I thought his heart arteries had narrowed, and he agreed to undergo a few studies. I obtained some blood tests that afternoon to see if his cholesterol or blood sugar were too high or if there were any other blood problems. In addition, I gave him a treadmill test. He was only able to walk on the treadmill for about five minutes before he began having chest pain. I glanced at the monitor. His EKG had clearly become abnormal, indicating that the pain was due to poor blood flow to the heart. By the time we got him off the treadmill, he was complaining of moderately severe chest pain, which we were able to relieve by placing some nitroglycerin under his tongue. This young man had a serious problem—one that required immediate intervention.

The next day, Jim went to the Cardiac Catheterization Laboratory for a coronary angiogram. (For more information on this test, see Chapter 11.) I watched as my colleague Dr. Alan Yeung, director of the Stanford Cardiac Catheterization Laboratory, skillfully threaded a coronary catheter up through Jim's femoral leg artery, up the aorta to the heart arteries. I kept an eye on the X-ray screen as Alan injected contrast dye into the heart arteries. What we saw was not pretty. There was an old blockage in one of the heart arteries that had caused the mild heart attack three years earlier. But now Jim had a new problem: one of his three main heart arteries was 90 percent narrowed by an angry-looking ulcerated plaque. Alan left the patient's side and walked casually back to the observation area where I was viewing the case. We spoke briefly. Alan wanted to proceed immediately; he could make the vessel wider using a balloon catheter, and then put in a metal stent to hold the vessel open. I explained the procedure to Jim as he lay on the table, and he agreed to let us go ahead with it. Alan reinserted the catheter with the stent and the procedure went smoothly. The final angiogram revealed Jim's right heart artery to be as good as new. It was lucky that he had listened to his wife and come to see us before the coronary artery occluded. That would certainly have resulted in a crippling heart attack and possibly death.

We sent Jim home the next day with instructions to take one baby aspirin daily, to continue the beta-blocker, to start a new cholesterol-lowering medication, and to follow my program for endothelial health. He is doing well, back at work and enjoying life.

Jim's tale sounds like a success story, but in some ways it is a failure. It is likely that Jim could have avoided a trip to the Cardiac Catheterization Laboratory at the age of 38. If he had taken preventive steps years before, he might have avoided our expensive and potentially dangerous intervention. He could have helped his body heal itself.

What exactly was going on inside Jim's blood vessels while he smoked, ate, sat, and worried? What was happening inside his body?

The very same lifestyle issues that put Jim at risk for cardiovascular disease also impaired his endothelium—and made him more susceptible to the disease of the blood vessels known as hardening of the arteries, or atherosclerosis, the buildup of plaque that narrows blood vessels. (Atherosclerosis comes from the Greek *athero,* meaning "gruel" or "paste," and *sclerosis,* meaning "hardness.")

As it is, in the course of normal life, we all do many things that destroy the health of our blood vessels, over and over again, sometimes without even realizing it. Jim's lifestyle is an example of this; he had many risks for cardiovascular disease and endothelial damage—family history, smoking, weighing too much, stress, sedentary lifestyle.

Unfortunately, Jim's problem is not an isolated case. It is symptomatic of what's going on all around us. The next time that you are in a public place in the U.S. or Europe, take a look at the people around you. Realize that half of the people you see are going to die from a heart attack or stroke. These two diseases are the biggest killers in the Western world, responsible for more deaths than any other causes combined. In addition to being the major killer, many more people suffer from the pain and limitations brought on by narrowed arteries. Some people have chest pain and shortness of breath. Others have pain in the legs when walking. All are at risk for becoming another heart disease statistic.

What Puts You at Risk for Atherosclerosis?

RESEARCHERS NOW believe that atherosclerosis is caused when the endothelium becomes dysfunctional. We know that the same conditions that put you at risk for developing atherosclerosis first impair the endothelium.

Most risk factors can be divided into two groups: those you can do something about, either by changing your lifestyle or taking medications; and those that you have no control over. What are these risk factors? And how do they weaken the endothelium?

RISK FACTORS THAT YOU CAN DO SOMETHING ABOUT

High cholesterol. Blood cholesterol level is a well-known risk factor for endothelial impairment and atherosclerosis. It is estimated that about 100 million Americans have high cholesterol. Is it any wonder—with the high amounts of saturated fat and cholesterol in our U.S. diet? Foods rich in animal fat—like fatty meats, whole-fat dairy products, and fried foods—are the biggest culprits.

We have known that cholesterol plays a role in cardiovascular disease since the 1960s. Since then, we've learned how to effectively lower cholesterol through diet and medication. We have powerful cholesterol-lowering medicines that prevent heart attack and stroke and save lives. Doctors now have very specific guidelines regarding how low cholesterol levels should be, depending on an individual's other risk factors. Unfortunately, some patients are not getting the right treatment. In Chapter 11, you will learn more about intensive care for the blood vessels of people with heart disease.

Smoking. Tobacco smoke has about 4,000 different substances in it, any number of which can contribute to adverse effects on the blood vessels. Even passive smoke (exposure to the cigarette smoke of someone else) damages blood vessels and accelerates plaque formation. Tobacco smoke contains a number of poisons, including nicotine, that harm the blood vessels. In my laboratory at Stanford, we have shown that nicotine can cause plaques and tumors to grow much more quickly. (*Short-term* use of nicotine patches or gums to stop smoking is safe).

Obesity or overweight. Excess body fat strains the heart, raises blood pressure, and boosts cholesterol levels. It also increases the risk of developing diabetes. People who are overweight tend to have higher blood pressure, higher blood sugar levels, and a more sedentary existence, all of which damage the endothelium.

Diabetes. This "silent epidemic," characterized by high blood sugar levels, seriously increases your risk of developing cardiovascular disease. When there are excess amounts of sugar in the blood, the sugar sticks to the proteins in the blood vessels. These "glycosylated" proteins do not function normally, nor does the body recognize them. Instead, the body's immune system thinks that these proteins are foreign and may attack them. The resulting inflammation in the vessel wall can damage the vessel and accelerate hardening of the arteries. Fortunately, vascular problems can be prevented or delayed with aggressive control of blood sugar.

Hypertension or high blood pressure. This disorder, caused by excessive pressure of the blood against the walls of the blood vessels and heart, strains both the heart and the blood vessels, causing damage over time. High blood pressure may be due to high levels of circulating hormones such as angiotensin and adrenaline. These are "stress" hormones that are useful to you if you are in a flight-or-fight situation. But if these hormones are chronically increased, they cause blood vessels to contract and raise blood pressure. Moreover, they cause blood vessels to make free radicals that damage the endothelium and reduce production of nitric oxide.

Sedentary lifestyle. People who are sedentary are twice as likely to succumb to a heart attack or stroke than people who are active. Daily exercise benefits cardiovascular health in a number of ways. Exercise reduces your bad (LDL) cholesterol, increases your good (HDL) cholesterol, reduces your blood sugar, reduces your stress hormones (adrenaline), reduces your resting heart rate and blood pressure, reduces your weight and has direct beneficial effects on your endothelium and blood vessels. In addition, you don't have to be an ultramarathoner to benefit from exercise; even moderate daily exertion (vigorous walking for 30 minutes daily) can add years to your life.

Homocysteine. Homocysteine is a modified amino acid that comes from another amino acid, methionine. Our bodies can make methionine, and we ingest it in the protein we eat. In a chemical reaction that is important to cell function, methionine is converted to homocysteine. However, high levels of homocysteine damage the endothelial cell. The most common cause of elevated homocysteine levels is vitamin B deficiency. Replacement of B vitamins can reduce homocysteine, and L-arginine or antioxidants like vitamin C may reverse the effects of homocysteine.

Stress. Stress takes its toll on the blood vessels. Like other muscles in the body, blood vessels contract and expand in response to the nervous system. Fear, anxiety, and stress can activate the nerve fibers of the blood vessels, releasing adrenaline-like substances into the vessel wall, causing it to relax or constrict. This explains how emotion can trigger angina when individuals have blood vessels narrowed by plaque. The emotional stress activates the nerves in the blood vessels, causing them to constrict.

The vasoconstrictor nerves that are activated by anger or other strong emotions also stimulate the adrenal gland to release adrenaline into the blood stream. Adrenaline makes the heart race. It also constricts vessels in the skin and gut and relaxes vessels to the heart and brain (to redirect blood to where it's needed in a fight-or-flight situation). Adrenaline also enhances the ability of the blood to clot. This is an appropriate reaction if you encounter a saber-toothed tiger, but not if you are caught in a traffic jam.

The parasympathetic nerves are the ones that slow the heartbeat and cause blood vessels to relax and open. Obviously, if you had a choice, you would prefer that these nerves have a greater influence over your coronary arteries and heart. The goal behind stress reduction is to tip the balance in favor of these parasympathetic nerves.

RISK FACTORS THAT YOU CAN'T DO ANYTHING ABOUT

Family history. The strongest risk factor for heart disease is a family history of heart attack or stroke at an early age (before the age of 55). Unfortunately, children of parents with heart disease are more likely to develop it themselves. As we learn more about genetic causes of heart disease through such research as the Human Genome Project and the Donald W. Reynolds Cardiovascular Clinical Research Center at Stanford University, we will identify new hereditary risk factors.

We already know about some of these hereditary risk factors. One of these is lipoprotein (a), a substance similar to low-density lipoprotein cholesterol (LDL, or bad, cholesterol), except that it is stickier and more likely to accelerate blood clot and plaque formation. Another hereditary risk factor is high blood levels of homocysteine. (See above.)

If you have a family history of premature hardening of the arteries, you should be tested for homocysteine and lipoprotein (a), because the treatment for these risk factors is quite specific. The treatment for high homocysteine levels is B-vitamin supplements, and the treatment for high lipoprotein (a) is high-dose niacin and antioxidant therapy. Antioxidants may also be useful in fighting high Lp(a) levels. Statins don't lower Lp(a), but by lowering LDL cholesterol, statins reduce the risk of elevated Lp(a).

Gender and age. While it is generally believed that men have a greater risk of heart attack than women—and have heart attacks earlier in life—women are also at risk after they go through menopause. Because women seem to have a 10-year lag before they succumb to vascular problems, many people may have the false impression that women do not have as much problem with heart attack and stroke. Nothing could be further from the truth. After menopause, women begin to catch up to men in terms of heart disease. As it turns out, the major cause of death in women is not breast, ovarian, or uterine cancer; it is heart attack and stroke. In fact, a woman who has a heart attack at an early age (around 50) is more likely to die during this event than a man of the same age.

Why are premenopausal women protected from these risk factors? We used to believe that estrogen was the answer. However, trials of estrogen therapy in postmenopausal women have been disappointing. Estrogen replacement does not seem to protect postmenopausal women from heart attack or stroke. Instead, premenopausal women seem to have another important survival advantage—namely, they make more NO than men of the same age. As women enter menopause, they lose this advantage, and postmenopausal women make the same amount of NO as men of the same age. It is very likely that the loss of protective NO is the reason why, after menopause, women begin to die from heart attack and stroke.

A Common Thread

WHY IS it that such seemingly unrelated factors—high cholesterol, high blood sugar, high blood pressure, smoking, sedentary lifestyle, and obesity—all lead to the same endpoint? What is the common thread that explains why each of these conditions can increase your risk of heart attack and stroke? You guessed it: lack of nitric oxide. Each of these risk factors injures the endothelium and reduces the production of nitric oxide, thus weakening your self-defense mechanism against heart attack and stroke.

Here is how the damage occurs.

ATHEROSCLEROSIS—A PROCESS THAT OCCURS THROUGHOUT YOUR LIFE

HARDENING OF the arteries begins very early in life, but luckily takes a long time to develop. By the time we are toddlers, the surface of our blood vessels already have small yellowish irregularities. These fatty streaks are minor blemishes on the surface of the blood vessel and present no immediate danger. In many civilizations, these blemishes do not progress any further. However, in societies where there is high consumption of animal fat, excess food intake, exposure to tobacco, and lack of adequate exercise, the process continues. By the time we are in our teens and young adulthood, most of us have well-established fibrous plaques in the arteries to our heart, head, and limbs. Although the fibrous plaques are not harmful, they are harbingers of bad things to come. If we persist in an unhealthy lifestyle, we will develop the third stage of this disorder, characterized by complex lesions, full-fledged atherosclerotic plaques that narrow the vessel and disturb blood flow. When they block 50 percent or more of the vessel, they restrict the amount of flow through the vessel and can begin to cause symptoms: chest pain, leg pain, or stroke. Unfortunately, by the time we are adults, this self-destructive process is already well under way and our vessels are beginning to thicken and narrow. But atherosclerosis is a slow and insidious process. It takes decades of an unhealthy lifestyle before there is a significant amount of plaque narrowing the vessel.

WHY PLAQUE FORMS—A NATURAL DEFENSE GONE AWRY

WE NOW know that atherosclerosis begins when the endothelium becomes injured or unhealthy. The endothelium loses its smooth, nonstick surface and instead becomes like cellular Velcro, pulling in white blood cells. These white blood cells, or monocytes, move from the blood into the vessel wall, where they become cells that attack and ingest the cholesterol that has accumulated in the vessel wall.

The question that has puzzled researchers until now is this: why do white blood cells move to the vessel wall and ingest fat? Scientists may now have the answer: they suspect that the process that causes atherosclerosis is similar to that involved in fighting an infection—except that instead of fighting a germ or bacteria, the white blood cells turn against another foreign invader, oxidized cholesterol in the vessel wall.

Cholesterol itself is not bad. In fact, it is essential for life. Cholesterol is a building block for all cell membranes. It is also the precursor for sex hormones and other steroids that our bodies manufacture. It is only when cholesterol becomes oxidized that the trouble begins. Here's how it happens.

When people eat and absorb fat, it goes into the bloodstream but doesn't float around freely. Instead, it is carried around in the bloodstream by proteins called lipoproteins. As most everyone knows by now, there are two types of lipoprotein. One type carries cholesterol to different parts of the body, including the artery wall; this type, the bad guy, LDL, low-density lipoprotein, causes problems when it carries too much cholesterol to the vessels. The other type, the good guy, HDL, high-density lipoprotein, carries cholesterol away from the vessel wall and eventually out of the body.

The roots of atherosclerosis can be traced to LDL cholesterol and its run-in with the vessel wall. Much of the action takes place within the endothelium itself.

High cholesterol (and other risk factors) make the endothelium sticky. As you now know, each of the risk factors impairs the ability of the endothelium to make NO. When the endothelium makes less NO, it becomes less like Teflon and more like Velcro.

In the meantime, cholesterol circulating in the blood gets trapped beneath the endothelium—and becomes oxidized there. Oxidized cholesterol is a foreign material to the body; it is perceived to be an invader, something that must be removed.

A fatty streak forms. In their effort to fight the enemy, the white blood cells adhere to the now sticky endothelium and penetrate into the vessel wall. There they gobble up the oxidized cholesterol. The problem occurs if you continue to eat a diet high in fat and processed foods. More cholesterol gets into the blood, and then into the vessel. The white blood cells continue to do their job, attacking and gobbling up the cholesterol. Eventually, the white blood cells in the vessel wall become grossly swollen with fat and turn into foam cells (so called because all of the fat in these cells give them a foamy appearance). Fearing that the oxidized LDL cholesterol is overcoming them, the foam cells send out signals of distress in the form of chemokines (proteins that lure and attract white blood cells). The foam cells also make the free radical known as superoxide anion in a misdirected attempt to destroy the invader. This only causes more problems because the superoxide anion further oxidizes the cholesterol that has accumulated in the vessel wall—and destroys NO. The result of all this misdirected effort is the formation of a fatty streak.

Plaque develops. Fatty streaks, which form yellowish blemishes on the vessel surface, do not disturb blood flow. But the foam cells in these blemishes can rupture through the endothelium. In the area of endothelial damage, platelets stick in an effort to seal off the tear. These platelets, along with the foam cells and injured endothelial cells, make growth factors that cause vascular smooth muscle cells and fibroblasts to migrate into the area. In an attempt to wall off the invasion, these cells make scar tissue around the fatty accumulation in the vessel.

Third-stage complex plaque forms. When the plaque becomes large and full of cells and debris, it is known as a complex plaque. Like an abscess or pustule in the skin, complex plaque consists of a fibrous cap that overlies an inner core of debris. The complex plaque protrudes beyond the inner surface of the vessel, into the vessel lumen (the space inside the vessel through which blood flows), obstructing the flow of blood (similar to the top of a pimple that protrudes beyond the surface of the skin). This domelike cap is composed of scar tissue, overlain by a thin layer of damaged endothelium. Underneath the dome is an inner core of gruel, similar to pus, made of liquefied cholesterol, crystals of calcium, dead cells, and the white blood cells that were trying to clean up the debris. (The process of cell death associated with an influx of white blood cells is called necrosis, which is what causes the formation of pus in an area of infection and inflammation.)

There is yet another similarity between complex atherosclerotic plaque and an abscess; eventually, they both may rupture. But the result of plaque rupture within a blood vessel is catastrophic; in fact, it is what causes the sudden onset of heart attack and stroke. What happens is this: white blood cells may invade the fibrous cap and begin to chew away the scar tissue, undermining and weakening the cap. With the stress of blood pressure and blood flow, the plaque ruptures, releasing the pus and causing blood to clot on the plaque. The clot blocks the vessel and the unfortunate individual suffers a heart attack (if the plaque was in the coronary artery), a stroke (if the plaque was in a carotid artery), or sudden onset of severe pain in the gut or leg (if the affected vessel happens to supply blood to the intestines or to the leg).

Besides rupturing, plaque may suddenly grow larger and cause a sudden onset of painful symptoms or even a heart attack. Although most plaque tends to grow slowly over the years, plaque may expand rapidly when microscopic vessels grow into the plaque, bringing more white blood cells. The plaque has now grown out well into the lumen of the artery and it is exposed continuously to the force of flowing blood. This barrage of pulsating blood flow strains the fibrous cap and the small microvessels within the plaque. Under the strain, these small vessels within the plaque may burst and release blood into the plaque, causing it to expand rapidly.

Your Ability to Reverse Plaque

WE USED to think that hardening of the arteries was an inevitable consequence of aging. We know now that this is not true. Plaque growth can be halted and even reversed. Research at Stanford and other institutions has shed light on the cellular mechanisms that are responsible for this disease. This knowledge is significant because as we develop a better understanding of this process, we can develop new therapeutic strategies to prevent, or even reverse, atherosclerosis.

Atherosclerosis is not like rusty deposits clogging the pipes or gobs of grease plugging the drain. It is like the Great Barrier Reef, a living thing, beautiful in its complexity. And like the reef, it may appear inanimate, but it is full of living cells and can change its shape and thickness.

At the microscopic level of individual cells, it is clear that atherosclerosis is a dynamic process that we can accelerate, turn off, or even reverse by the lifestyle choices we make. Atherosclerosis is a cellular defense mechanism gone awry; a number of different cells and proteins share the blame with cholesterol and the other risk factors.

The endothelium, overlying the dome of the complex plaque, serves as a barrier or as a welcome mat to other cells passing by in the bloodstream. Its role—as barrier or welcome mat—depends on its health. When it is healthy, it is not sticky. However, when it's unhealthy—because of tobacco use, sedentary lifestyle, diabetes, or high blood pressure—it is sticky, attracting white blood cells that litter its smooth surface. These cells enter and migrate through the plaque, ingesting fat and cell debris in an attempt to clean up.

Each of the cells is capable of influencing another one's behavior. Cells make and release proteins and other substances that can cause their neighbors to grow and multiply or shrink and die. The activity and behavior of these cells can cause plaque to grow larger or to regress, to become quiet and stable, or, like a microscopic volcano, to become volatile and erupt with catastrophic consequences.

The point: the plaque in your vessel wall is not a lump of lard. It is alive. This is good news, because a living thing can be influenced in its behavior. With the therapeutic strategy that I will outline in later chapters, you will be able to restore the health of your endothelium and influence the behavior of these cells so as to prevent the growth of plaque. Furthermore, you will be able to cause preexisting plaques to regress. Most important, you will be able to transform the menacing complex plaque filled with lipid and necrotic debris to a more stable fibrous plaque that is less likely to rupture and cause problems in the future. In addition to decreasing the size and volatility of the plaque, I will show you how you can restore the ability of your vessels to relax normally and therefore accommodate more blood flow to critical organs such as your heart.

HOW DO RISK FACTORS CONTRIBUTE TO ATHEROSCLEROSIS?

What about the other risk factors for heart disease? How do they figure into the picture? In the first place, you have to have elevated cholesterol to develop atherosclerosis. But the other risk factors contribute by impairing the endothelium and reducing the influence of

NO. Risk factors also increase the generation of free radicals by the vessel, causing the cholesterol in the vessel to become oxidized, which incites the invasion of white blood cells.

DO BACTERIA OR VIRUSES PLAY A ROLE IN ATHEROSCLEROSIS?

The resemblance of atherosclerosis to an infection has caused investigators to ask if bacteria or viruses might be involved in the development of atherosclerosis. Interestingly, a form of atherosclerosis that affects pigeons is caused by a virus (Marek's virus). Bacteria and virus particles have been found in human plaque and are more likely to be found there than in normal vessels. Some studies have found an association between certain infections, such as *Chlamydia pneumoniae*, herpes simplex, and cytomegalovirus (CMV), and the chance of having a heart problem. These germs could potentially cause an inflammatory response in the vessel that could accelerate atherosclerosis. There are studies under way to see if, by reducing infection with antibiotics, risk of heart attack or stroke is also reduced. We have recently found that CMV causes endothelial cells to generate enormous amounts of ADMA. Although the bacteria/virus hypothesis is interesting, it remains unproven.

HOW THE WHITE BLOOD CELL GOES ASTRAY (AND THE DEVELOPMENT OF ATHEROSCLEROSIS)

To help you visualize how white blood cells fight oxidized cholesterol, let's become a white blood cell in the battle.

A white blood cell is small, but is two to three times larger than a red blood cell. There is a good reason why we are bigger; we have a different job than the red blood cell. Instead of bringing oxygen to the body, we are policemen, continually on the prowl for foreign invaders. It is our job to search out and destroy these invaders.

Let's say the endothelium becomes injured and its adhesion molecules grab onto us while we are floating around the bloodstream. We white blood cells stick to the endothelium and penetrate through it and into the vessel wall. Once there, we find ourselves gobbling up oxidized LDL cholesterol, the perceived enemy.

As long as blood cholesterol is high and in the vessel wall, we continue to stick to the endothelium and infiltrate into the vessel so as to gobble up oxidized LDL cholesterol—until we are grossly swollen with fat.

At this point, we are called a foam cell. Fearing that oxidized LDL cholesterol is winning the battle, we send out distress signals to the chemokines (proteins that lure and attract more of us). We make the free radical, known as superoxide anion, in a misdirected attempt to destroy the invader. But this only causes more problems for the vessel wall because the superoxide anion further oxidizes the cholesterol.

The destruction process is well under way. In response to the oxidative stress caused by the superoxide anion that we are releasing, the endothelium makes more adhesion molecules and chemokines to attract more of us. And more cholesterol is oxidized in the vessel wall. The superoxide anion also destroys the NO that is usually there.

Again, we white blood cells play a role in the rupture of plaque. The plaque looks like an abscess to us. We decide to get rid of the debris by popping the abscess. Therefore, we invade the fibrous cap overlying the debris in the plaque. We begin to chew away the cap, undermining and weakening it. With the stress of blood pressure and blood flow, the plaque ruptures, releasing the pus and causing blood to clot on the plaque. The result of this plaque rupture is a heart attack or stroke.

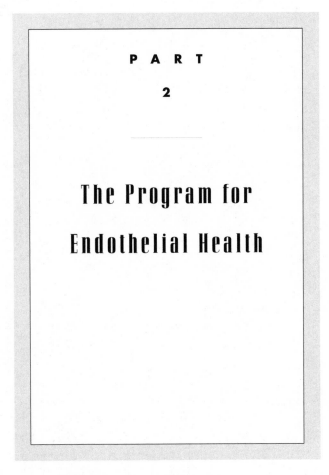

P A R T

2

The Program for
Endothelial Health

Chapter 4

Eating to Enhance NO—
the Diet: Principles That Last a Lifetime

Your Endothelium Knows What You Eat

JUST ONE fast-food meal can make your endothelial cells sick. Even if you are otherwise healthy, one fast-food meal reduces the ability of your blood vessels to function normally for several hours.

This rapid decline in endothelial function was first observed by Dr. Robert Vogel at SUNY.[1] Using ultrasound to view relaxation of the arm artery, Dr. Vogel studied people before and after a meal—a hamburger and french fries—loaded with saturated and trans fat. Study participants were healthy young people with normal endothelial function and no risk factors for atherosclerosis. Two hours after eating the fast-food meal, participants had an increase in blood fat levels, and their endothelial function deteriorated to about half of normal. In subsequent studies, Dr. Vogel showed that the adverse effects of a fast-food meal can be prevented by eating certain nutrients, such as antioxidants.

The implications of these studies are significant. An unhealthy meal immediately damages the endothelium. If you regularly bombard your endothelium with this kind of meal, you may cause long-term damage to your vascular system.

But just as you can harm the endothelium with a poor diet, you can restore its health with a good one. Here is where my diet comes in. As you'll see, it's especially designed to maintain the health of the endothelium—to improve blood flow, reduce symptoms of cardiovascular disease, and prevent heart attack and stroke.

WHAT DOES THE ENDOTHELIUM SEE WHEN YOU EAT?

What does the endothelium see when you digest different types of food?

• When you eat carbohydrates, the endothelium sees sugar (whether you've eaten a vegetable or a cookie). When the carbohydrate is in the form of white bread or pasta, the endothelium just sees sugar. But when the carbohydrate is in the form of fruit, the endothelium sees sugar as well as other heart-healthy nutrients such as vitamins, antioxidants, and phytochemicals.

• When you eat fat, the endothelium sees the fatty acids, depending on the type of fat you've eaten. If you eat a french fry, the endothelium sees saturated and trans fatty acids. However, if you eat nuts, the endothelium sees monounsaturated (good) fatty acids, as well as vitamin E and other plant nutrients.

• When you eat protein, the endothelium sees the individual amino acids from the protein source. If you eat a Big Mac, the endothelium sees a mixture of amino acids that includes more methionine (the amino acid that is the precursor for homocysteine, which can damage the endothelium). If you eat soy protein, the endothelium sees a mixture of amino acids that includes more L-arginine (which is good for the endothelium) as well as other phytochemicals that help endothelial function.

Maintaining a Healthy Weight

CARRYING THE appropriate amount of weight for your height and frame is a very important aspect of vascular health. Why? If you are overweight, your body has an increase in stored lipids or fat tissue. People who are overweight also tend to have high blood cholesterol, blood sugar, and blood pressure. All of these conditions damage endothelial tissues. Shedding just a few pounds can markedly improve each of these conditions and put you on the road to a healthier cardiovascular system.

How will you know if you are overweight? You can determine whether you need to lose a few pounds by using the body mass index (BMI). The BMI, a standard measure of healthy weight, is based on the ratio between your height and weight. (BMI is your weight in kilograms divided by the square of your height in meters.) The chart makes it easy for you to calculate your BMI; all you need to know is your height and weight. Using the chart on page 50, locate your height in inches in the left-hand column, and then find your weight in the corresponding row. Your BMI is the number, between 19 and 35, at the top of the column where your height and weight intersect.

If your BMI is between 21 and 25 kg/m²:

Good work! You are at a healthy weight—and you'll want to keep it that way. My diet and exercise plan will help you stay healthy.

If your BMI is between 26 and 29 kg/m²:

You need to adhere to my diet and exercise plan so that you can achieve a healthy BMI. Following my diet and exercise program, you will lose about one to three pounds per month. Don't expect to lose more. If you lose too much in one two-week period, the weight is likely to come back as quickly as you lost it. It is better to change your lifestyle, maintain these changes, and lose weight gradually. That way, the excess weight will be gone forever.

If your BMI is at or greater than 30:

You need to follow my program. However, you may also need to see a dietitian who will supervise a weight loss program for you.

Body Mass Index

To use the table, find the appropriate height in the left-hand column labeled Height. Move across to a given weight. The number at the top of the column is the BMI at that height and weight. Pounds have been rounded off.

BMI	19	20	21	22	23	24	25	26	27	28	29	30	31	32	33	34	35
Height (inches)	Body Weight (pounds)																
58	91	96	100	105	110	115	119	124	129	134	138	143	148	153	158	162	167
59	94	99	104	109	114	119	124	128	133	138	143	148	153	158	163	168	173
60	97	102	107	112	118	123	128	133	138	143	148	153	158	163	168	174	179
61	100	106	111	116	122	127	132	137	143	148	153	158	164	169	174	180	185
62	104	109	115	120	126	131	136	142	147	153	158	164	169	175	180	186	191
63	107	113	118	124	130	135	141	146	152	158	163	169	175	180	186	191	197
64	110	116	122	128	134	140	145	151	157	163	169	174	180	186	192	197	204
65	114	120	126	132	138	144	150	156	162	168	174	180	186	192	198	204	210
66	118	124	130	136	142	148	155	161	167	173	179	186	192	198	204	210	216
67	121	127	134	140	146	153	159	166	172	178	185	191	198	204	211	217	223
68	125	131	138	144	151	158	164	171	177	184	190	197	203	210	216	223	230
69	128	135	142	149	155	162	169	176	182	189	196	203	209	216	223	230	236
70	132	139	146	153	160	167	174	181	188	195	202	209	216	222	229	236	243
71	136	143	150	157	165	172	179	186	193	200	208	215	222	229	236	243	250
72	140	147	154	162	169	177	184	191	199	206	213	221	228	235	242	250	258
73	144	151	159	166	174	182	189	197	204	212	219	227	235	242	250	257	265
74	148	155	163	171	179	186	194	202	210	218	225	233	241	249	256	264	272
75	152	160	168	176	184	192	200	208	216	224	232	240	248	256	264	272	279
76	156	164	172	180	189	197	205	213	221	230	238	246	254	271	271	279	287

How to Maintain a Healthy Weight

EXERCISE IS one way to help you lose or maintain a healthy weight. But it is not sufficient on its own.

Just as the right diet is crucial to vessel health, so is portion size—or, in other words, calorie control, how much you eat. One of the secrets of eating a healthy diet is sticking to portion sizes. If the menu calls for a half cup or five ounces, don't use one cup or eight ounces. It may sound obvious, but it's not always easy to do. Keeping portion size on track requires discipline and attention to detail. But, like anything else, if you practice, if you do it enough, it will become natural to you.

As for portion size, think small or medium rather than large, extra large, or supersize. On all packaged foods, use the Nutrition Facts panel to determine the amount of one serving and the size of that serving.

Here are some rough guidelines for different types of food:

Vegetables and potatoes	1 cup is about the size of an average-sized fist
Fish or chicken (or meat)	1 portion is about 3 ounces or the size of a deck of cards

Use these guidelines to help you gauge or estimate portion sizes. There is no one portion size that is right for everyone. (Note that the portion sizes in my menus and recipes vary slightly.) However, in order to shed any unwanted pounds, you must keep an eye on your calorie intake and practice healthy serving size control.

As for calories, my diet is designed around a calorie level of about 1,800 calories a day—which will result in weight loss for those who need to lose weight and will help those at ideal body weight maintain their weight. About 1,500 to 1,800 calories a day is a low-calorie diet for any adult. But anyone who needs to lose weight will do so on this diet, particularly when it is combined with the exercise program. Even if you are not overweight, this diet will help you maintain your healthy weight. Remember, though, that the focus of the program is to eat a healthy diet and take care of your endothelium, not to count calories.

Principles of the Diet

THE PRINCIPLES of my diet are based on nutritional and cardiovascular science. In designing this diet and lifestyle program, we used an evidence-based approach that is sadly lacking in many popular diet books. (Evidence-based means that every recommendation made is based on rigorous scientific study.)

The studies upon which this diet is based include investigations of endothelial function and nutrition from my lab and others; the Lyon Diet Heart Study (a Mediterranean diet); and the DASH study (which emphasizes low fat, fruits and vegetables, and whole grains). Both the Lyon Diet Heart Study and the DASH study have been scientifically tested and found to be successful dietary interventions to prevent cardiovascular disease (Lyon diet) and to reduce high blood pressure (DASH study). To develop my diet, we incorporated lessons from each of these studies with new data regarding nutrition and endothelial health. My diet is best described as a *modified* Mediterranean diet. But before we discuss the modifications, let's review the components of a Mediterranean diet and why it's so good for cardiovascular health.

THE MEDITERRANEAN DIET

THE INITIAL Lyon Diet Heart Study was conducted in France between 1988 and 1992. In this landmark study, researchers compared a Mediterranean-style diet to a standard low-fat diet (based on the low-fat American Heart Association diet recommended at that time). Researchers studied the impact of these two diets in participants who had survived a first heart attack. The Mediterranean-style diet consisted of an increased intake of fresh fruit and vegetables, whole grain cereals, vegetable protein (legumes), antioxidants, minerals, folate, B_6, and omega-3 fatty acids and fish. Some of the differences in the diet? As you'll see in the chart below, the Mediterranean diet has higher levels of good types of fat—including polyunsaturated, monounsaturated, and omega-3—less cholesterol, and more fiber.

THE LYON DIET HEART STUDY

How the two diets compared—the Mediteranean diet versus a standard low-fat diet:

	Mediterranean Diet % of calories	Standard Low-Fat Diet % of calories
Total fat	30	34
Saturated fat	8	11
Polyunsaturated fat	5	6
Monounsaturated fat	13	11
Omega-6 fatty acids	3.6	5.3
Omega-3 fatty acids	0.84	0.29
Cholesterol	203 mg	312 mg
Fiber	18.6 g	15.5 g

The Lyon study was terminated after 27 months because the cardiovascular health of participants on the Mediterranean-style diet improved greatly. Researchers found that these study participants had a noticeable reduction in heart attacks during the study. Even four years later, in a follow-up study, researchers observed that those on the Mediterranean-style diet reduced their chances of suffering another heart attack by 50 to 70 percent. The conclusion to both the initial and follow-up studies: dietary changes can protect us from heart disease.

The big question is then, of course, what are the essential elements of this protective diet? The secret goes beyond the amount of fats, carbohydrates, and proteins, and involves the types and sources of these nutrients. The Mediterranean diet is so named because it is similar to the diet of people living near the Mediterranean Sea. Researchers knew from studies such as the Seven Countries Study, conducted in the 1960s, that the death rate from heart disease in southern and central European countries adjacent to the Mediterranean Sea—Spain, France, Italy, Portugal, and Greece—was one-third to one-fourth that of other European countries such as Scotland, Ireland, the Czech Republic, Finland, and Hungary. In contrast to the diet of northern Europeans who eat more flour, sugar, and refined foods, the Mediterranean diet generally consists of vegetables, fruits, grains, fish, and beans.

As described in *The Lancet* in 1994, the diet recommended in the Lyon Diet Heart Study consisted of less saturated fats, cholesterol, and linoleic acid, and more oleic and alpha-linolenic acid. (See beginning p. 61 for information on these types of fats.) The dietary changes made by the group eating a more Mediterranean-type diet included the following:

- more whole grain bread
- more root and green vegetables
- more fish and less meat (red meat was replaced with chicken)
- more fruit
- replacement of butter and cream with canola oil and olive oil for salads and food preparation

In comparing both diets, many researchers concluded that one of the most notable distinctions between the diets was the higher amount of polyunsaturated oils—namely, omega-3 fatty acids—that may have played a role in lowering the risk of cardiovascular disease. This led researchers to suspect that omega-3 fatty acids may have contributed to the protective effects of the diet.

THE DASH STUDY

THE DASH (Dietary Approaches to Stop Hypertension) study is a research project funded by the National Heart, Lung, and Blood Institute and conducted by the Brigham and Women's Hospital, the Center for Health Research in Portland, Duke University Medical Center, Johns Hopkins University, and Pennington Biomedical Research Center in Louisiana.

The study, which was designed to determine the effect of diet on blood pressure, found in 1997 that the DASH diet lowered blood pressure. The study found that the diet was as strong as any single medication in reducing blood pressure in patients with hypertension.

The DASH diet consists of lots of vegetables, fruits, and low-fat dairy products, and is low in both fat and saturated fat. In a follow-up study, the diet lowered salt intake by limiting processed foods high in sodium. The researchers suggested techniques to keep sodium intake down (to no more than 2,400 milligrams a day): using spices, herbs, and fruit juices to season food; rinsing canned vegetables to remove excess salt; and limiting salty foods such as ham and other cured meats, pickles, vegetables in brine solutions, and canned ready-to-eat foods such as soup.

Components of My Diet

MY DIET is a modified Mediterranean diet, and combines the best of the DASH and Mediterranean diets, with some additional twists based on new insights in research about what makes the endothelium healthy. The diet emphasizes a variety of whole foods, including nuts, seeds, beans, legumes, whole grain breads and cereals, and fruits and vegetables. There is an emphasis on nutrient-dense foods that are high in L-arginine, omega-3 fatty acids, and phytonutrients such as antioxidants and phytoestrogens. Arginine-rich protein sources are emphasized, including fish, nuts, legumes, and soy products.

This balance of L-arginine-rich proteins, nutrient-dense carbohydrates, and healthy types of fat provides maximal blood lipid protection from oxidation; helps to maintain blood glucose and insulin in the normal range; and offers adequate amounts of key vitamins for a heart-healthy diet. The diet also boosts NO production and enhances endothelial health. And it does all this in as little as two weeks (remember how quickly the endothelium responds to what you eat). In addition, the diet includes both familiar foods that will enable you to follow the diet easily and effortlessly, as well as new ways to cook and prepare foods such as soy.

The diet provides:

- 30 percent of calories from fat, replacing saturated fats with mono- and polyunsaturated fats from foods such as nuts, fish, and canola and olive oils
- 20 percent of calories from protein, maximizing the L-arginine content of protein foods such as soy, beans, nuts, chicken, and fish
- 50 percent of calories from carbohydrates, with an emphasis on whole grains, nuts, legumes, fruits, and vegetables—foods that contain phytonutrients, nutrients from plants that provide protective benefits and that nutrition scientists are only just beginning to identify and appreciate

This calorie breakdown is unusual in several ways:

- It allows more dietary fat intake than some diets for heart health—replacing saturated fats with omega-3 fatty acids, and mono- and polyunsaturated fats.
- It encourages fiber intake, in amounts greater than those of the typical American diet.
- It discourages processed foods that are high in salt, saturated and trans fats, and nutrient-empty calories.
- It is rich in phytonutrients that have antioxidant properties, as well as those that improve vascular relaxation.
- It promotes foods that are high in L-arginine levels.

Another aspect of my diet is the recognition that some individuals, particularly those with symptoms of heart disease, benefit from dietary supplementation in addition to a healthy diet. The role of dietary supplementation is discussed in detail in Chapter 10.

HOW IS THIS DIET DIFFERENT FROM OTHERS?

MY DIET

My diet is designed for people with heart disease or for those at risk of heart disease. It is a healthy and tasty diet that provides 30 percent of calories from fat (mono- and polyunsaturated, the good kinds); 50 percent of calories from carbohydrates (enriched with plant fiber); and 20 percent from protein (largely plant-based or fish proteins, which are loaded with antioxidants, phytochemicals, and L-arginine). My diet has a scientific basis, and each of its components has been shown to benefit the health of the heart and blood vessels. Rich in plant-based carbohydrates and vegetable protein that are known to reduce blood pressure, the diet is rich in fiber, which lowers cholesterol and helps to reduce weight by making you feel full. It utilizes lots of soy protein since people who eat more soy protein have less chance of a heart attack. The diet helps you lose weight slowly, and keep it off, particularly when combined with the exercise program. My diet is similar to the American Heart Association (AHA) Step I diet, except that it is higher in soy protein, fiber, phytonutrients, and arginine and lower in cholesterol. It is slightly more liberal in total fat than the AHA Step II diet (30 percent versus 20 percent fat), but provides for the same amount of saturated fat (about 7 percent of calories).

HIGH-PROTEIN DIETS

Compare the high-protein diets[2]:

	Protein	Fat	Carbohydrates
Atkins	27 percent	68 percent	5 percent
The Zone	30 percent	·30 percent	40 percent
Stillman	64 percent	33 percent	3 percent

High-protein diets are high in protein and fat. You can rapidly lose weight on a high-protein diet because they change your metabolism (metabolic ketosis), which reduces hunger. Unfortunately, these diets are also high in animal protein, which is high in methionine and harmful to your endothelium. Animal protein does not contain the fiber and phytonutrients that are so beneficial to the metabolism and blood vessels. Animal protein is also high in saturated fat, which impairs your endothelium. There is no evidence that a high-protein diet will help you if you have heart disease. In fact, there is evidence that a high-protein diet can harm you if you have heart disease. A typical high-protein meal at a fast-food place impairs your endothelium within hours. It is no wonder, then, that epidemiological studies have shown that people who regularly consume high amounts of red meat (such as people following the Atkins diet) are twice as likely to have a heart attack or stroke. High-protein diets may also increase your chance of getting gout, osteoporosis, and (if you have diabetes) kidney disease.

ULTRA-LOW-FAT DIETS

Diets such as the Ornish or Kurzweil diets demand a reduction in fat to 10 percent of total calories. Dr. Ornish's treatment for patients with heart disease is a total regimen: a vegetarian diet with less than 10 percent of calories from fat and minimal amounts of saturated fat (the "Reversal Diet"); moderate exercise (usually a walking program), daily use of stress-management techniques, group support and psychological counseling, and a smoking cessation program. In contrast to the advocates of high-protein diets, Dr. Ornish has done the hard work of testing the effects of his regimen. He has demonstrated that this total program can slow and even reverse coronary artery narrowings. In a follow up study of 48 patients in his Lifestyle Heart Trial published in *Journal of the American Medical Association,* Dr. Ornish found fewer cardiac events in people on his program. The Multicenter Lifestyle Demonstration Project, published in the *American Journal of Cardiology,* followed 333 patients with symptomatic coronary artery disease on the program; 77 percent improved so much that they no longer required surgery. It is not clear which parts of the treatment—diet, exercise, group support, counseling, stress reduction, or smoking cessation—are responsible for the benefit. The reduction in fat to 10 percent of calories is very demanding and is essentially a vegetarian diet that many people just can't tolerate for a long period of time. There is evidence that an ultra-low-fat diet causes problems in people with insulin resistance syndrome (high triglycerides, low

HDL cholesterol, and higher insulin levels). Low-fat, high-carbohy-drate diets like the Ornish diet typically increase triglyceride (blood fat) levels and lower HDL (good) cholesterol. In our Vascular Clinic at Stanford, we have seen people on the ultra-low-fat diets with high triglycerides and low HDL cholesterol; these individuals actu-ally improve their cholesterol levels when we have them modestly increase the fat in their diet. There is also some evidence that very-low-fat diets might increase the chance of stroke. Nevertheless, it seems likely that for certain people the ultra-low-fat diet may be use-ful. For people with coronary artery disease and high LDL (bad) cholesterol, *particularly those who do not have low HDL cholesterol and high triglycerides*, ultra-low-fat vegetarian diets may be a rea-sonable alternative to the diet recommended in this book.

Making Food Choices

DISTINGUISHING BETWEEN FATS

DIETARY FAT has gotten a bad reputation. So much so that some people have gone too far to cut fat out of their diet, replacing it with unhealthy levels of refined carbohydrates. We need some fat to maintain tissues inside the body, as well as healthy skin.

Fat is an essential component of every cell in our body. Our cells also need vitamins that are found only in fat: the fat-soluble vitamins A, D, E, and K. In addition, essential fatty acids linoleic and linolenic (omega-6 and omega-3) are necessary for health—and are available to us only in the foods we eat.

So fat is not something you want to do without. But the truth is that all dietary fats are not the same. Remember that I'm not talking about calories here. All fats, no matter the type, contain the same amount of calories (about 9 calories per fat gram). But some fats are simply healthier for your cardiovascular system than others. My diet recommends that you get 30 percent of your calories from fat—with an emphasis on healthy fats. There's nothing wrong with eating di-etary fat—as long as you're careful about the type you eat.

What's the main difference between fats? There are basically two different groups of fats: saturated and unsaturated. Both are made up of a chain of carbon and hydrogen molecules. In saturated fat, the carbon atoms are "saturated" with hydrogen atoms—they have as many as they can hold. In unsaturated fats, on the other hand, the carbon atoms are not filled up with hydrogen. In both polyunsaturated and monounsaturated fats, there are fewer hydrogen atoms (there is at least one unsaturated bond, one place where a hydrogen atom could be added).

You can see the difference between saturated and unsaturated fats. The more saturated the fat, the harder it is at room temperature. Butter contains the most saturated fat. By contrast, margarine has more polyunsaturated fat and is softer. Oils have the most polyunsaturated fat and are liquid. The more liquid the fat, the better it is for your heart and vessels.

The type of fat we eat even affects our cells. Fats are an essential part of the membrane that surrounds every cell in our body. When the cell membrane has more saturated fat in it, it becomes stiffer. When the cell membrane has more mono- or polyunsaturated fat in it, the cell membrane becomes more flexible. As you can imagine, we want our cells to be flexible, not stiff. Flexible cells can circulate through your blood vessels easier. Also, flexible cells are more responsive to signals throughout your body. For example, when endothelial cells are exposed to saturated fat, they are not as responsive to blood flow. On the other hand, when they are exposed to unsaturated fat, they are more flexible and responsive to the flowing blood.

AVOIDING SATURATED FAT AND TRANS FATTY ACIDS

IN ADDITION to making your cells less flexible, there are other problems with saturated fat. For a long time now, we have known that saturated fat (fat from animals) raises blood cholesterol levels to a greater degree than does unsaturated fat. In fact, what most people may not realize is that blood cholesterol levels have more to do with the amount of saturated fat you eat than with the amount of cholesterol you eat.

Besides saturated fat, the other type of fat that you will want to avoid is called trans fatty acids. This type of fat is often found in processed foods, including commercially baked goods such as crackers, cookies, cakes, pretzels, and potato chips, for example. Trans fat, which is composed of trans fatty acids, is made by manufacturers when they harden liquid vegetable oil to turn it into a solid (as in a stick of margarine). This occurs when manufacturers add hydrogen to unsaturated fats, making them more like saturated fats. (Generally the harder the margarine or vegetable shortening, the more trans fat is included in the product.)

The nutrition label of the product doesn't list trans fat as an ingredient in the product. The nutrition label mentions instead that the product contains partially hydrogenated oil. If you see this on the nutrition label, you can be assured that the product contains trans fat (since partially hydrogenated oil is a common form of trans fat). For the manufacturer, this process protects the product against spoilage and preserves flavors. But for your blood vessels, there is no advantage at all. This type of fat raises blood cholesterol levels. Partially hydrogenated fats are similar to saturated fats because they raise blood levels of bad cholesterol (LDL), but not the levels of good cholesterol (HDL). In a study conducted in the Netherlands, researchers found that men who consumed the most trans fatty acids (6.4 percent of total calories) had twice the risk of developing heart disease than those who consumed the least amounts (2.4 percent). Because of publicity about its dangers, consumption of trans fatty acids has decreased in the Netherlands. Americans get about 2 percent of their calories from trans fatty acid, while western Europeans ingest as little as 0.5 percent. In the near future, federal agencies in the U.S. may require manufacturers to indicate how much trans fat is in a product. Meanwhile, avoid products that have partially hydrogenated vegetable oil.

GET TO KNOW THE GOOD FATS

SO WHAT type of fat do you want to eat? My diet encourages you to choose a mix of polyunsaturated and monounsaturated fats.

All oils and fats are mixtures of different types of fat (for example, canola oil is an excellent oil that contains both polyunsaturated and monounsaturated fat). Different foods, too, can contain different types of fat. For example, one serving of avocado (one-fifth of a medium one) contains 5 grams of fat, of which 1 gram is saturated, 3 are monounsaturated, and 1 is polyunsaturated. As a general rule, the amount of saturated fat in vegetables and fish tends to be lower than the saturated fat from animals. (Note that our recipes include very small amounts of saturated fat; when you do use butter, make sure you use a very small amount; or better yet, replace the butter with one of the plant sterol margarines described in Chapter 10.)

Monounsaturated Fats

Monounsaturated fats (sometimes referred to as omega-9s or oleic acid) are good fats that come from plants. They are found in olive oil, canola oil, and certain peanut oils (and some foods such as avocado, nuts, and olives).

Monounsaturated fats reduce LDL (bad) cholesterol in the blood and have no effect on HDL (good) cholesterol. Keeping in mind that many oils and foods contain a mixture of different fats, some of the most common sources of monounsaturated fats are some nuts and nut oils, such as almonds, hazelnuts, and pecans. (The Adventist Health Study, published in 1992, found that consumption of nuts greatly reduces the risk of fatal and nonfatal heart disease.)

Polyunsaturated Fats

Polyunsaturated fats are also good fats, and include the omega-3 and omega-6 fatty acids. In chemistry the Greek letter omega (Ω) is a symbol of the double bond between carbons in the carbon chain of the fatty acid. The number refers to the position in the molecule in which the first double bond occurs: for example, in omega-9, the first double bond occurs after nine carbons; in omega-6, six carbons in; and in omega-3, after the third carbon in the chain.

Both omega-3 and omega-6 fatty acids are considered essential dietary components, which means that humans are incapable of producing them on their own. Neither omega-3 nor omega-6 fatty acids contribute to an increase in blood cholesterol levels. By contrast, trans fatty acids contribute, as do saturated fatty acids, to an increase in blood cholesterol levels.

The Omega-6s

Omega-6 fatty acids (linoleic acid) are polyunsaturated fats that are found in vegetable oils such as corn, safflower, soybean, and sunflower oils. It is generally believed that omega-6s lower blood levels of LDL (bad) cholesterol, as well as HDL (good) cholesterol.

The Omega-3s

Omega-3 fatty acids have been found to have an anti-inflammatory effect (which is beneficial in heart disease since the process of atherosclerosis involves inflammation of the vessel wall). Although the primary source of omega-3 comes from fish, some plants are also rich in omega-3, including some nuts, dark leafy vegetables, and flaxseed (an especially rich source of omega-3, since 55 percent of its oil is linolenic acid).

The marine omega-3 fatty acids, found in the oils of fish, are very beneficial. In 1980, two Danish physicians, Drs. Bang and Dyerberg, published a remarkable observation regarding Greenland Eskimos.[3] They found that despite the fact that Eskimos eat a very-high-fat diet that includes whale blubber, they seldom have heart attacks or strokes. In fact, their chance of having a heart attack is only about one-tenth that of the average American. Why doesn't the fatty diet of the Eskimos lead to heart problems?

The answer is in the fat itself. The Eskimo diet is almost entirely derived from fish and other marine animals. As it turns out, the fat in fish is different from the fat in other animals and has beneficial effects on the heart and blood vessels.

About 40 percent of the fatty acids in fish are omega-3 polyunsaturated fatty acids, specifically eicosapentaenoic acid (EPA) and docosahexaenoic acid (DHA). These omega-3s have several heart-healthy attributes. Besides keeping the cells themselves flexible, they also make our vessels more pliable, and thereby make the work of the heart easier.

Omega-3s also improve endothelial function. They enhance the production of NO, thus improving blood vessel relaxation. Also, omega-3s can be used by the body to make a form of prostacyclin. Like NO, prostacyclin relaxes blood vessels, improves blood flow, reduces thickening of the vessel, and prevents blood clots. Omega-3s also interfere with the production of thromboxane, a substance that can cause blood vessels to constrict and platelets to clot. It is not surprising, then, that researchers have found that fish oil supplementation can improve relaxation of blood vessels in people with hardening of the arteries and can reduce the chance of blood clots forming in the vessel.

Fish oil also has favorable effects on blood cholesterol levels, increasing the good (HDL) cholesterol and reducing the bad (LDL) cholesterol. Fish oil, which is helpful in reducing triglycerides in the blood, also reduces the body's production of free radicals and substances that cause inflammation. As we discussed earlier, inflammation of the blood vessels contributes to hardening of those vessels. Inflammation also affects common joint and skin diseases; by suppressing inflammation, fish oil has been shown to help alleviate the joint pain of arthritis and to improve eczema and psoriasis.

GETTING THE MOST OMEGA-3S FROM FISH AND OTHER FOODS—WHAT TO CHOOSE

Although all fish and seafood contain some omega-3 fatty acids, some fish have greater amounts than others. Fish with the highest content of omega-3 tend to be fatty, cold-water fish such as mackerel, salmon, and trout.

What is the best source of omega-3s, farmed or wild fish? Nutrition scientists continue to debate this point. And, in essence, it seems to depend on the type of fish. For example, when salmon and trout are farmed, they require a diet of other fish in order to survive and grow. So farmed salmon and trout are similar to their wild counterparts in terms of omega-3s. Farmed catfish, on the other hand, can survive on a diet of grains—which may explain why farmed catfish typically does not contain omega-3s.

FISH WITH HIGHEST OMEGA-3 FATTY ACID CONTENT

(Grams per 100 grams of food)

Mackerel	5.3
Herring	3.1
Salmon	2.0
Trout	1.6
Sardine, canned in oil	1.3
Halibut	0.9
Swordfish	0.8
Surimi	0.6
Shrimp	0.5
Catfish	0.4*
Fast-food fish sandwich	0.4*
Fish sticks	0.4*
Crab	0.3
Cod	0.3
Clams	0.3
Plaice	0.2
Haddock	0.2
Flounder	0.2

Tuna, canned in oil	0.2
Pike, northern	0.1

* However, in these products, the fat is oxidized by frying so that there is minimal or no "good" fat.

VEGETABLES WITH HIGHEST OMEGA-3 FATTY ACID CONTENT

(Grams per 100 grams of food)

Flaxseed	22.8
Walnuts, English	6.8
Soybeans, roasted	1.5
Wheat germ	0.7
Beans, dry	0.6
Almonds	0.4
Avocado	0.1

Sources: www.nal.usda.gov/fnic/foodcomp/Data/index.html and *American Journal of Clinical Nutrition* 71 (2000 supplement): 179S–88S.

How much fish should you eat? Most of us would benefit from increasing fish intake in our diet. Approximately one serving (about three to six ounces of fish) several times a week is ideal. Follow the menu pattern in the diet for guidance on increasing fish in your diet.

Whenever you eat fish, be sure that it is broiled or baked rather than fried, since frying adds excess fat, some of which is oxidized. (And oxidized fat is very bad for your blood vessels.)

BALANCING THE OMEGAS

MOST EXPERTS agree that we get enough omega-6 fatty acids in our diet. But we fall short on the omega-3s. Currently, the ratio of linoleic (omega-6) to linolenic acid (omega-3) in the modern diet is about 20:1. It would be better if the ratio were between 10:1 and 5:1. The menu plans here ensure that you get the right balance of omega-3s and omega-6s.

POWERFUL PROTEINS

THE WORD *protein* comes from the Greek word meaning "of prime importance." Proteins are present in foods, as well as in tissues in our bodies. They are composed of amino acids, the body's building blocks. Proteins are broken down during digestion into amino acids that the body then uses to grow and repair tissues. There are about 22 amino acids (or building blocks) that the body needs. Together, these amino acids make up thousands of different proteins in the body—proteins that include hormones, antibodies, and enzymes.

Protein is a component of many tissues and functions within the body. For example, one type of protein, keratin, is the major building material for hair, skin, and fingernails. Other proteins include hemoglobin (carries oxygen in the blood); insulin, a hormone (regulates blood sugar); and certain structural proteins (such as those involved in muscle contraction) and plasma proteins (such as those involved in blood clotting). Proteins also play an important role in maintaining heart and vessel health. One of the proteins that helps maintain cardiovascular health is NO synthase, a particular type of protein that is also an enzyme. (Enzymes speed up chemical reactions. NO synthase speeds up the conversion of L-arginine to NO.) When a particular protein (such as those above) is broken down, the body must make a new one, precisely modeling it on the previous one. To do this, your body must have a source of each amino acid.

Essential amino acids, of which there are at least nine, cannot be made by the body in significant quantities. They must come from the foods we eat. Protein foods contain various combinations of these amino acids. The nonessential amino acids are also important, but they can be made in the body and thus are not necessary to obtain through diet.

In some people, a nonessential amino acid can become essential. (You need to get it from the foods you eat.) That is sometimes the case with L-arginine. For example, depending on an individual's health, L-arginine can be essential. In times of physiological stress, intense exercise, or trauma, L-arginine can become, as nutritionists call it, "conditionally" essential. Under these conditions, your body will not be able to make sufficient L-arginine, and you will have to get some from your diet. In times of health, your body can make enough L-arginine. However, in people with risk factors, there may be a relative deficiency of L-arginine due to high levels of ADMA. Even in healthy people, the levels of L-arginine in the body are partially dependent on how much you take in through diet.

HOW PROTEINS STACK UP

LIKE FATS, not all sources of protein are created alike. In general, vegetable protein (for example, soy and beans) is better for you than animal protein because it contains no saturated fat and less methionine (which converts to homocysteine, which can injure your endothelium). In addition, vegetable proteins also have more phytonutrients and fiber than do animal sources.

Some protein sources are "more complete" than others. A complete protein source is a food that contains all nine essential amino acids in quantities that are similar to those needed by the body. Incomplete proteins are those that lack sufficient amounts of one or more essential amino acids. Proteins from animals—milk, fish, poultry, meat, and eggs—are considered complete proteins. For a long time, proteins from plants were considered incomplete. But then researchers found that soy protein is an exception to the rule.

Today, nutritionists have analyzed exactly how protein foods stack up in terms of their amino acid content as well as other factors. The Protein Digestibility-Corrected Amino Acid Score (PDCAAS) has become the current standard by which protein foods are measured, recognized by both the FDA and the Food and Agricultural Organization working jointly with the World Health Organization. The PDCAAS assesses several factors—a protein food's amino acid content, its digestibility (how easy it is for your body to break down the protein and absorb it), and its ability to supply essential amino acids in amounts adequate to meet human needs. The highest value a protein food can have is 1.00—and the egg white takes its place as the leader. A few years ago, researchers determined that soy protein (soy protein isolate, the most concentrated form of soy) also has a score of 1.00.

THE AMINO ACID SCORE

Protein Source	Protein Digestibility Corrected Amino Acid Score
Soy protein isolate*	1.00
Casein	1.00
Egg white	1.00
Beef protein	.92
Pea flour	.69
Kidney beans (canned)	.68

Pinto beans (canned)	.63
Rolled oats	.57
Lentils (canned)	.52
Whole wheat	.40
Wheat gluten	.25

Source: "Protein Quality Evaluation, Report of the Joint FAO/WHO Expert Consultation." FAO Food and Nutrition Paper No. 51, 1989 (FAO/WHO 1991).

* Value for soy protein isolate provided by Protein Technologies International.

Although most vegetable proteins have a lower amino acid score, by combining them you can easily get to 1.0. Beans and rice complement each other well. So do other combinations of legumes and grains. If you eat a variety of vegetables, you can get all the amino acids you need. And as mentioned above, if you eat soy protein, you get all of the amino acids you need. *And vegetable protein is a much better source of amino acids because you also get fiber and phytonutrients that you do* not *get when eating animal protein.*

My diet is designed so that you get 20 percent of your calories from protein, maximizing the L-arginine content of protein foods. The menus feature many dishes with soy, beans, nuts, chicken (without the skin), and fish. Egg whites are also a good source of protein. (People should limit their intake of egg yolks, because they are high in cholesterol.) Soy is a wonderful source of protein and also contains other substances that are healthy for your blood vessels. When soy is mentioned, most Americans think only of tofu. Tofu is made from soy—and is a good source of protein—but there are many other ways to eat soy protein. (See Some Soy Favorites on p. 70.)

L-ARGININE

L-ARGININE IS a semi-essential amino acid found in certain protein foods. (As I explained above, it is essential or nonessential depending on your body's needs.) Beans, legumes, nuts, fish, soy, and chicken are all good sources of protein—and are high in L-arginine. (Red meat and eggs are also high in L-arginine. However, we do not recommend the consumption of red meat and egg yolk. They are high in cholesterol and saturated fat and do not contain the high amounts of fiber and other nutrients available in plant sources of L-arginine.)

The average American adult takes in 1 to 4 grams of L-arginine daily. (Unfortunately, most of this—about 75 percent—comes from red meat.) Although healthy individuals get enough L-arginine from dietary sources, those with symptoms of heart or vessel disease may benefit from more L-arginine, as much as 6 to 9 grams of L-arginine daily—too much to get from diet alone. (See Chapter 10 for information on dietary supplements.)

PROTEINS WITH B VITAMINS (FOLATE, B$_6$, AND B$_{12}$)

IT'S IMPORTANT to eat foods packed with B vitamins. Among other benefits, B vitamins help keep your vessels healthy; they also keep the body's homocysteine levels low and prevent endothelial injury.

The most common cause of elevated homocysteine levels is vitamin B deficiency and low dietary levels of B vitamins—namely, folate, B$_6$, and B$_{12}$. Many protein foods contain the vitamins B$_6$ and B$_{12}$, which can lower homocysteine. Good sources of B$_6$ are navy beans, walnuts, salmon, and chicken. Poultry, fish, and shellfish (especially clams and oysters) contain B$_{12}$. Furthermore, plant protein contains less methionine than animal protein; therefore, eating more plant and less animal protein helps maintain healthy homocysteine levels in the blood.

GO FOR SOY

SOY IS an excellent source of protein. It is a complete protein and has components that have been found to promote heart and blood vessel health. Soybeans are a rich source of the phytoestrogens known as daidzein, genistein, and glycitein. (Phytoestrogens are estrogenlike substances that come from plants.) These soy phytoestrogens, also called isoflavones, have been shown to have a variety of benefits: they can help reduce symptoms of menopause such as hot flashes; they may protect against prostate and certain breast cancers; and they can provide a variety of benefits to the cardiovascular system. (The only caveat about soy products: they contain a fair amount of oxalate, as do spinach, rhubarb, and beet greens.[4] Oxalate increases calcium excretion in the urine. For this reason, these vegetables should be eaten in limited quantities by people who have kidney stones.)

Although there has been a lot of confusion about the value of these natural estrogenlike substances, there is a substantial amount of research that indicates that men and women who consume more plants that contain phytoestrogens have fewer heart attacks and strokes and reduced rates of cardiovascular risk factors and coronary disease. The Japanese, for example, have half the cardiovascular disease of Americans; their protection from heart attack and stroke may be due to their high consumption of soy.

New and exciting unpublished research from my group at Stanford has also found that in postmenopausal women with high cholesterol, daidzein and genistein have a dramatic ability to improve vessel relaxation, by a completely different mechanism than L-arginine. We found that a daily pill containing daidzein and genistein improves the ability of the blood vessels to respond to nitric oxide. In addition to helping the vessels relax, genistein and daidzein have been found to be anti-inflammatory agents as well as antioxidants, able to soak up the free radicals that cause damage to blood vessels.

Soy can also reduce cholesterol levels. When cholesterol levels are high, daily intake of soy protein (25 to 50 grams or one to two servings of soy protein powder) can reduce total cholesterol and LDL (bad) cholesterol, as well as triglycerides, by about 10 percent. (If cholesterol is already at a healthy level, soy will not reduce it further.) In fact, even the Food and Drug Administration now permits the claim that 25 grams of soy protein can lower cholesterol when taken in conjunction with a diet low in saturated fat and a healthy lifestyle.

In our studies at Stanford, we found that capsules containing 50 milligrams of phytoestrogens (a mixture of purified daidzein and genistein, with a small amount of glycitein) taken daily markedly improved vasodilation. (This is equivalent to the amount of phytoestrogens in 50 grams of soy protein.) Although phytoestrogens are milder than estrogen (they have only about 1/1000th the activity of estrogen), consuming a diet high in soy protein can raise levels of phytoestrogens in the blood to a point where they benefit blood vessel health.

As you'll see, our menus demonstrate many different ways to get more soy into your diet—from using soy to make "jam" and as a replacement for egg, sour cream, and cheese, to using it in the old favorite campfire dessert, s'mores. (See recipes for Apricot Spread, p. 96; Red Lentils with Beets and Tofu "Feta," p. 150; Soy'mores, p. 160; and others.)

REGULAR OR SILKEN TOFU: WHICH SHOULD YOU BUY?

There are two types of tofu: regular and silken. Both come in three textures: silken, firm, and extra firm. Regular tofu, particularly the extra firm kind, is chewy and holds together well during cooking. It can easily be cut into small pieces for stir-fry and can be marinated. Silken tofu, on the other hand, contains a lot of water. Pureed, it is good in dips, dressings, soups, and desserts. In cooking, even firm silken tofu breaks apart in stir-fries.

SOME SOY FAVORITES

Here are some of my favorite ways of getting soy into the diet:

- Edamame, the soybean steamed in the pod, has a mild, slightly sweet flavor (similar to sweet peas). It's a great side dish or snack. Or add the edamame beans to a salad.

- Textured soy protein (TSP) in bite-size pieces is another favorite. (I like So Soya's.) TSP is convenient because it has a long shelf life and doesn't need refrigeration. Use it in stir-fries. (It has a texture and taste that resembles chicken.)

- Soynuts are small, crunchy kernels that have a grainy taste. By themselves, they are not very exciting. I add them to a combination of dried fruit, fresh fruit, and/or nuts. I often eat a bowl for breakfast, dessert, or as a snack.

- Soymilk, soy yogurt, and soy cereals are all good choices. Be on the lookout for soy products that have added sugar and fat because these products will not make your heart healthier. Just because a product contains soy doesn't mean it is good for your heart. For example, soy sauce has a lot of salt in it. Read the label of soy products carefully.

MORE SERVINGS OF WHOLE GRAINS, FRUITS, AND VEGETABLES

CARBOHYDRATES ARE more than just potatoes and rice. Whole grains, fruits, and vegetables all contain carbohydrates (as well as varying degrees of proteins and fats). All carbohydrates supply energy to the body and fuel the central nervous system. Whether present in food as sugars or starches, carbohydrates are all broken down into sugar (glucose) and are carried through the bloodstream to fuel our cells. My diet provides 50 percent of calories from this type of food. But, as with fat, the question is what kind is best, what kind is most packed with nutrients?

MEETING DAILY REQUIREMENTS WITH NUTRIENT-RICH CARBOHYDRATES

LIKE FATS, all carbohydrates are not equal. The nutrient value of fruits, nuts, vegetables, beans, and whole grains is much higher than that of any type of refined or commercially prepared food. Our diet relies on carbohydrates that are full of nutrients. Studies have shown that regular consumption of whole grains, fresh fruit, and vegetables prevents death from stroke and heart disease because they lower blood pressure (based on the DASH study) and because they contain nutrients that keep your endothelium healthy. For example, antioxidants in fresh fruits and vegetables can preserve NO from destruction; isoflavones can increase the synthesis of NO; L-arginine can make NO; and other nutrients can help make cofactors for the synthesis of NO.

THE POWER OF WHOLE GRAINS

HAVE YOU ever wondered why whole wheat bread is better for you than bread made from refined flour? We just assume that whole wheat is better without questioning why. The reason refined flour (and white bread) is not as good for you is that most of the nutrients are lost in the refining process. When wheat is refined, the bran (or outer shell) of the grain is removed. Some of the nutrients lost in refining are replaced, and that's why flours and breads are labeled "enriched." But not all nutrients lost in refining are replaced.

What exactly is a whole grain? Whole grains and products made from whole grain contain all parts of the grain. This includes the bran or outer shell that contains the fiber and nutrients.

It's important to read labels carefully when selecting whole grain products. Many products that claim to be made of multigrains are full of refined grains that have no added nutrient benefit. To ensure that a product has whole grains, look for wheat, oats, corn, or rice as the first ingredient in the list. You will know it is whole grain if the words *whole* or *whole grain* appear before the grain's name in the ingredient list. In a study of about 34,000 Norwegians, researchers at the University of Minnesota found that those who ate the highest amounts of whole grains had a 23 percent reduced risk of death from heart disease compared to those who ate lesser amounts or no whole grains.

HOW FIBER IMPROVES ENDOTHELIAL HEALTH

ANOTHER REASON that whole grains are better for you is that they contain more fiber. Fiber is found only in plants, including beans, legumes, nuts, fruits, vegetables, and whole grains. Most of it passes through the body without being digested. There are two different types of fiber: soluble and insoluble, and each plays a different role in the body. Just as some fatty foods contain different types of fat, foods with fiber contain a mix of soluble and insoluble fiber.

Soluble fiber absorbs water. Certain grains and plants, such as oatmeal, barley, beans, oat bran, nuts, legumes, pectin (from fruit), and psyllium, contain soluble fiber. Many studies have shown that soluble fiber can lower blood cholesterol levels, which will also help to improve endothelial health.

Insoluble fiber does not mix with water. It is found in whole wheat goods, seeds, nuts, and wheat bran. Insoluble fiber is also available in the skin of fruits and whole vegetables. Insoluble fiber, on the other hand, does not affect cholesterol levels. Insoluble fiber can help in weight reduction or weight management since it slows down the digestive process and the rate at which your stomach empties, helping you to feel full longer.

When you eat more fiber, you should also remember to drink water to maintain healthy hydration; most people should drink more water during the day, which improves both the digestion and elimination processes. It's generally recommended that you drink about eight 8-ounce glasses of water daily, although all fluids (except alcohol) count toward the total. (Although coffee, tea, and soda can contribute, it is not wise to depend solely on these beverages for your fluid intake.)

THE BENEFITS OF FRUITS AND VEGETABLES

I RECOMMEND that you eat seven to nine servings of fruits and vegetables daily. Why fruits and vegetables? Fruits and vegetables are nutrient-dense foods; compared to other foods, the body gets many more nutrients than calories from them.

Fruits and vegetables contain many, many phytonutrients and are loaded with antioxidants, including carotenes (vitamin A or beta-carotene), tocopherols (vitamin E compounds), ascorbate (vitamin C), and polyphenols (molecules that have several carbon rings and are very effective at detoxifying free radicals). (See All About Polyphenols on page 74.)

There is much research supporting the anticancer properties of plant foods. Many of the findings also apply to cardiovascular medicine. For example, the antioxidant activity of many of the molecules in these foods reduces the risk of cancer and also reduces oxidative stress on the endothelium. Oxidative stress activates genes responsible for producing proteins such as the adhesion molecules and chemokines that change the endothelium from smooth and well-functioning to sticky and dysfunctional. The same antioxidants that fight cancer also stimulate the antioxidant enzyme glutathione S-transferase (GST), which preserves NO and fights cardiovascular disease.

Recently, nutrition scientists have discovered the various health benefits of the nonnutritive substances in plants known as phytonutrients or phytochemicals. Fruits and vegetables contain over 4,000 different phytochemicals that, working individually or together, appear to be good for your cardiovascular system. *Phyto* is Greek for "plant," and phytochemicals are plant chemicals. Those that enhance your endothelial function are typically antioxidants. We are just beginning to learn about the beneficial effects of these phytochemicals, including a host of flavonoids and carotenoids that protect your vessel from free radicals. Although some of these phytochemicals have been isolated and are available in pill or capsule form in health food stores, it is better for you to get these phytochemicals in their natural form. It is likely that there are important beneficial interactions between the phytochemicals in the fresh fruit or vegetable that would not exist in a processed supplement.

There is one fruit or juice that I ask my patients to avoid. Grapefruit, and grapefruit juice, interferes with the breakdown of many drugs. If you take any medication, grapefruit will probably interfere with the way your body handles the medicine. Accordingly, it is best to avoid grapefruit or its juice if you take medicine regularly. Have oranges or other citrus fruits instead.

ALL ABOUT POLYPHENOLS

Fruits and vegetables are loaded with about 4,000 different varieties of polyphenols. People who eat foods rich in polyphenols are less likely to have a heart attack or stroke.

There is a network of antioxidants in our body that includes enzymes (glutathione peroxidase, superoxide dismutase, catalase), small molecules (urate), and vitamins (tocopherols and tocotrienols that are forms of vitamin E; carotenoids, forms of vitamin A; and ascorbic acid, vitamin C). The polyphenols are needed for the proper and balanced functioning of this network. Polyphenols can prevent the oxidation of vitamin E and reduce the clumping of platelets.

Foods that are particularly rich in polyphenols include apples, blackberries, blueberries, cherries, citrus fruits, dark chocolate, grapes (white and red), lettuce, onions, persimmons, plums, potatoes, raspberries, red peppers, soy, strawberries, tomatoes, and wheat bran. Apples, blueberries, and cherries are the champions of the polyphenols, containing the highest amounts. Coffee, tea, wine, beer, and fruit juice also contain high amounts. (In fact, a glass of any of these has as much antioxidant activity as a glass of orange juice. The antioxidant activity of orange juice comes mainly from vitamin C rather than polyphenols.) Vegetables, legumes, and cereals have fewer polyphenols than fruit (this is particularly true of cereals made from refined flour, which contains negligible amounts of polyphenols).

Polyphenols are often lost in processed foods. For example, the peel of many fruits is enriched in polyphenols in comparison to the pulp (the peel also contains more fiber). This is also true of wheat, where the polyphenols are in the outer layers of the wheat grain, which are lost during refining of the flour.

Researchers have found that oxidative stress in the bloodstream goes up after eating a high-fat meal containing animal protein, while it goes down after a plant-based meal. One glass of red wine, which contains the polyphenols quercetin and resveratrol, has the same effect as 500 milligrams of vitamin C. (When you drink a glass of red wine while eating a fatty meal, it can blunt the adverse effect of the meal on your endothelium.)

The most common groups of plant antioxidants are the flavonoids (a type of polyphenol) and the carotenoids. Many flavonoids in plants (including fruits, vegetables, nuts, and whole grains) are antioxidants that protect LDL cholesterol in the blood from oxidation, stop platelet clumping, and have anti-inflammatory properties. Cruciferous vegetables (such as broccoli) are particularly enriched in flavonoids. So too are green tea and grapes. Indeed, some of the benefits of red wine have been ascribed to its flavonoid content. Resveratrol and quercetin are found in grape skin, grape juice, and red wine. (Unlike red wine, white wine is not fermented with the skin of the grape. It is the skin of the grape, and not the pulp, that contains most of the antioxidants.)

The color of fruit and vegetables is pleasing to the body, as well as to the eye. Plant pigments are another powerful source of healing. The carotenoids (including beta-carotene) give carrots and cantaloupe their orange color, and lycopene gives tomatoes its red color. Lycopene appears to be at least as potent as vitamin E as an antioxidant, and is best absorbed when the tomato is cooked.

Whole grains and nuts all contain phytochemicals, including polyphenols, terpenoids, pigments, and natural antioxidant vitamins such as vitamins A, C, and E. Grains contain phytonutrients such as plant sterols, phytases, phytoestrogens, lignans, and saponins, among others. These substances also have beneficial effects that may reduce the risk of cardiovascular disease. Fruits, vegetables, and certain grains also have isoprenoid compounds that are known to reduce total and LDL blood cholesterol.

FOODS AND THEIR PHYTONUTRIENT CONTENT

The following foods contain different types of phytonutrients that have been shown to benefit the heart and blood vessels:[5]

Food	Phytochemicals	Benefit
Garlic, onions, cabbage, broccoli, brussels sprouts, cauliflower	Sulfur compounds	Increases protective enzymes
Carrots, winter squashes, sweet potatoes, apricots, spinach, kale, parsley, cantaloupe	Carotenoids	Antioxidants
Most fruits and vegetables, flax, green tea, chocolate	Bioflavonoids	Antioxidants
Soybeans, beans, peas, peanuts	Isoflavones	Improves vessel relaxation
Mustard, horseradish, radishes, cruciferous vegetables	Indoles	Increases protective enzymes
Citrus fruits	Limonoids, terpenes	Antioxidants
Garlic, parsley, squash, basil, mint, eggplant, citrus fruits, tomatoes	Monoterpenes	Antioxidants
Broccoli, cabbage, soy, peppers, whole grains	Plant sterols	Reduces cholesterol
Oats, peas, beans, banana, apple, pear	Soluble fiber	Reduces cholesterol

GOOD NEWS FOR CHOCOHOLICS

There is a great deal of research that shows that small amounts of chocolate (particularly dark chocolate) can benefit the heart and blood vessels. Chocolate contains polyphenols similar to those in tea, fruits, and vegetables. These antioxidants reduce the oxidation of cholesterol and protect nitric oxide. Moreover, some of the polyphenols in chocolate also increase the production of nitric oxide. When people eat a chocolate bar, these polyphenols are absorbed and have been shown to increase the ability of the blood to protect itself against oxidative stress. Perhaps because of its effects on nitric oxide, chocolate consumption also reduces the clumping of platelets.

Chocolate as medicine is not a new concept. Centuries before the Spanish arrived, the native people of South America (the Olmecs, Mayas, and Aztecs) used chocolate to stimulate the appetite and to increase energy and alertness (our word for cocoa is derived from the Olmec *kakaw*). They used chocolate paste to mask the taste of bitter medicines.

If you are healthy, you don't need to feel guilty about occasionally eating chocolate (just use it in moderation, to avoid too many calories and saturated fat). I even allow my heart patients to consume small amounts of chocolate. However, chocolate does contain a caffeinelike substance that increases heart rate. Patients who have a problem with irregular heartbeats should limit chocolate for this reason (because tea and coffee also contain caffeine, they should also be avoided by people who have a problem with irregular heartbeats).

EAT FRUITS AND VEGETABLES LOADED WITH ANTIOXIDANTS, INCLUDING VITAMINS B, FOLATE, C, AND E

FRUITS AND vegetables are the best source of carbohydrates, because in addition to fiber they are loaded with micronutrients required for health. (Whole fruit is better than fruit juice because it contains more fiber.)

The micronutrients that are good for your heart and blood vessels include antioxidants (such as vitamins C, E, and beta-carotene), enzyme cofactors (substances that help enzymes to function, such as

B_6, B_{12}, and folate), and minerals (such as potassium, zinc, and magnesium). Like protein foods high in vitamin B, grains, legumes, green leafy vegetables, and root vegetables are also good sources of B vitamins that can lower homocysteine levels.

By consuming at least seven servings of fruit and vegetables daily (seven to nine are preferable), most people can obtain adequate amounts of the majority of these micronutrients and vitamins. (What exactly is a serving? It's one piece of fruit or a half cup of chopped or cooked fruit. It's one cup of raw vegetables or a half cup of cooked vegetables.)

GETTING NUTRIENTS FROM FOODS, NOT SUPPLEMENTS

AS YOU can see, fruits and vegetables, fish, nuts, whole grains, and legumes are just some of the foods that offer protection against cancer and heart disease. Because many of us don't eat seven to nine servings of fruit and vegetables a day, we could all improve our intake of them. Our two weeks of menus will help you see how to increase these foods in your daily meals.

What about supplements? Can you not worry about what you eat and get the nutrients you need from supplements? What about vitamins or fish oil supplements? In Chapter 10, you'll find out when supplementation can help. There is evidence that certain supplements can benefit people with symptoms of heart and vessel disease. However, for most healthy people who want to maintain their ideal body weight and stay healthy, the jury is still out on the benefit of taking supplements. It is not yet known whether consuming concentrated extracts of fruits and vegetables is advantageous. So far, though, researchers do know one thing: eating a diet rich in fruits, nuts, and vegetables will give you the benefit of a natural pharmacy of phytonutrients, which is the best protection against cardiovascular disease.

THE FRENCH PARADOX—COULD IT BE THE RED WINE?

The French Paradox is this: how is it that the French eat large amounts of fatty foods, yet have fewer heart attacks than other Europeans? Some of the clues to French cardiovascular health include types of foods consumed, such as fresh fruit and vegetables and less red meat. A possible contributing factor could also be the regular consumption of moderate amounts of red wine with meals.

Red wine is known to contain potent antioxidants such as resveratrol and quercetin that may enhance heart health. Indeed, researchers have shown that red wine (but not white wine) can cause vessels to relax in vitro. This relaxation is due to the protection of NO by the antioxidants in the wine—found mainly in the skin of the grape. This explains why red wine (which is incubated with the skin) has a stronger protective effect on the endothelium than white wine (which is not incubated with the skin). Actually, you don't need to drink red wine to get this effect; purple grape juice works just as well! Researchers in Boston have shown that consumption of three glasses of purple grape juice improves the ability of the blood vessels to relax in people with impaired endothelial function.

However, the benefit of red wine does not appear to be due solely to the antioxidants in the grape skin. Indeed, several large population studies have shown that one or two alcoholic drinks daily reduce your risk of heart attack, and it doesn't matter what form of alcohol is consumed. Researchers are still unclear about why these benefits occur, but they suspect several possible reasons: the blood-thinning property of alcohol, its ability to increase HDL (good) cholesterol, and the possibility that alcohol has an anti-inflammatory effect. Researchers in Germany found that, among 2,000 men and women, those who drank moderately had fewer signs of inflammation in the body compared with nondrinkers or heavy drinkers. Moderate drinkers had lower levels of C-reactive protein (CRP), a blood protein that is part of the body's inflammatory response. Some studies have noted that CRP levels are high in those at risk for heart disease. (Remember that inflammation plays a leading role in hardening of the arteries.)

One or two servings of beer, wine, or hard liquor daily appear to be good for you. In fact, you are better off than someone who doesn't drink at all. The benefit of moderate alcohol consumption even extends to people with diabetes. Studies have shown that people with diabetes who consume one drink daily have a reduced risk of death from heart attack or stroke in comparison to those who don't drink at all. However, it is important to point out that having more than two or three drinks daily can lead to other health problems. Heavy consumption of alcohol causes high blood pressure, irregular heartbeats, and sometimes even heart failure. The key? The saying is old, but true: "everything in moderation."

NUTRIENT/FOOD LISTS

HERE ARE SUGGESTIONS FOR SOME FOODS RICH IN THE FOLLOWING NUTRIENTS:

Vitamin A (Carotenoids)
Apricots
Cantaloupe
Spinach
Broccoli
Carrots
Sweet potatoes
Tomatoes
Winter
   squashes

Vitamin B$_{12}$
Fish
Milk (and milk
   products)
Eggs
Meat (an
   occasional

serving of very
   lean meat)
Poultry

B$_6$
Fortified cereals
Beans
Meat (an occasional
   serving of very
   lean meat)
Poultry
Fish
Some fruits and
   vegetables

Vitamin C
Broccoli
Oranges
Cantaloupe

Lemons
Peppers (sweet and
   hot)
Tomatoes
Citrus fruits

Vitamin E
Vegetable oils
Nuts
Leafy green
   vegetables
Fortified cereals
Wheat germ

Fiber
Blueberries
Carrots
Prunes
Raisins

Fiber (cont.)
Oranges
Sweet potatoes
Whole grain
    breads
Oatmeal
Bran flakes
All types of
    dried beans,
    legumes, and
    peas

**Folic Acid
    (Folate)**
Whole grain
    breads and
    cereals
Ready-to-eat
    cereals
Avocado

All types of dried
    beans, legumes,
    and peas
Oranges
Spinach
Strawberries

**L-Arginine-Rich
    Proteins**
All types of dried
    beans, legumes,
    and peas
Fish
Soy (tofu)
Egg whites
Meat (an
    occasional
    serving of very
    lean meat)
Chicken

Nonfat milk and
    milk products
Walnuts, almonds,
    peanuts, all nuts

**Polyunsaturated
    Fats**
Canola oil
Olive oil
Corn oil
Walnut oil
Avocado oil
Trans-free safflower
    margarine

Chapter 5

Making Food Choices—
Two Weeks of Menus (Including Recipes)

Y

OUR ENDOTHELIUM is unusual because its condition is very much based on what you eat. So you can imagine the obvious benefit after two weeks of healthy meals! These menus and recipes, which offer new food choices and new ideas about food preparation, will strengthen your endothelium. Let our two weeks of menus help you establish a healthy pattern of eating that you can continue for the rest of your life.

TIPS ON EATING OUT AND CONTINUING
THE HEALTHY PATTERN OF EATING

The menus and recipes are designed to give you a good example of healthy food-preparation techniques. You will find that as you become familiar with them, you will not only be able to select the healthiest recipes from your favorite cookbooks, but will also be able to apply the same pattern of eating, anytime, anywhere.

Here are a few ways to continue the healthy pattern of eating:

1. Stick to correct portion sizes. We all know that some restaurants serve whopping big portions. Don't feel as though you have to finish everything on your plate. Keep portion size in mind (re-

member the size of a deck of cards) and try not to overeat. Once you get accustomed to smaller portion sizes, it will be easier to stick to them. You'll find that you just won't be comfortable overeating.

2. Keep in mind the healthy types of fat while you are eating out. Fish (as long as it's not fried) is always a healthy choice, as are vegetables and fruit. Go easy on added fats: for instance, ask for salad dressing on the side so you can control how much you use; keep added fats, such as butter or sour cream, to about one tablespoon per meal.

3. Many ethnic foods are healthy. Japanese, Chinese, Thai, and even Mexican foods are full of healthy choices, including lots of fish, vegetables, rice, and legumes. At an Italian restaurant, healthier choices may include fish or pasta with vegetables, but beware of plentiful cheeses and creamy sauces.

4. Always choose foods that have been baked, poached, steamed, broiled, or grilled, as opposed to fried or deep fried.

5. Snacking on fruit, even dried fruit, is a much better bet than any prepared foods such as potato chips or cookies.

6. Make it easy for yourself to have healthy snacks. We stock up on dried fruits and berries, assortments of nuts, including soy nuts, and fresh fruit. In the morning, I will often throw a handful of nuts and dried fruit in a bowl, chop up some fresh fruit, and have a quick and healthy breakfast.

7. When choosing desserts, try to keep your fat intake to a minimum: sorbet, fruit cup, or frozen yogurt, for example. If you are going to splurge on a fancy, fattening dessert, try not to eat all of it.

Two Weeks of Menus

These menus are examples of healthy eating. You can also establish a lifetime of healthy eating by following the general recommendations in Chapter 4.

* Indicates a recipe.

DAY ONE

BREAKFAST

1 cup orange juice
1½ cups soy breakfast cereal with 1 tablespoon chopped almonds
1 sliced banana
8 ounces soymilk or low-fat dairy milk

LUNCH

Smoked Turkey Wrap with Dried Cranberries*
Celery and Edamame Slaw*
1 pear

DINNER

Linguini with Roasted Vegetable Sauce*
Mesclun salad with walnuts and Flax Vinaigrette*
Red Grape Macédoine*

Calories	1,785
Protein	62.1 g
Carbohydrates	282.3 g
Fiber	39.8 g
Fat Total*	56.0 g
Saturated	6.7 g
Mono	23.2 g
Poly	19.2 g
Cholesterol	43.9 mg
Arginine	4.1 g

* Please note that throughout the menus and recipes, saturated, mono, and poly grams combined may not equal total fat because of other fatty acid components in those foods that have not been analyzed here.

DAY TWO

BREAKFAST

1 cup orange juice
Muesli*

LUNCH

2 cups Butternut Squash, Chickpea, Tomato, and Corn Soup*
Romaine Salad with Shaved Parmigiano-Reggiano*
8 Whole Wheat Pita Crisps*
1 orange

DINNER

Turkey Meatloaf*
Broccoli with Roasted Garlic*
Brown Rice and Red Lentil Pilaf*
1 cup fresh berries
1 Soy'more*

Calories	1,873
Protein	78.3 g
Carbohydrates	270.5 g
Fiber	48.7 g
Fat Total	64.7 g
Saturated	11.6 g
Mono	28.6 g
Poly	13.5 g
Cholesterol	59.2 mg
Arginine	3.7 g

DAY THREE

BREAKFAST

1 orange, peeled and sliced
2 Pumpkin Muffins*

LUNCH

Tuna, Apple, and Arugula Salad*
2 Whole Wheat Crostini* with 2 teaspoons Herb-Infused Olive Oil*
1 cup Summer Fruit Salad*

DINNER

Red Pepper Stuffed with Barley and Black Beans*
Steamed kale with sesame seeds
1 cup Cherry Berry Compote* with ½ cup vanilla soy frozen dessert

Calories	1,804
Protein	62.7 g
Carbohydrates	250.4 g
Fiber	41.5 g
Fat Total	70.7 g
Saturated	9.7 g
Mono	31.9 g
Poly	15.7 g
Cholesterol	71.0 mg
Arginine	3.2 g

DAY FOUR

BREAKFAST

1 cup hot Irish oatmeal with 2 tablespoons
golden seedless raisins
8 ounces soymilk or low-fat milk

LUNCH

Black Bean Soup*
2 Tomato Bruschetta*
1 apple

DINNER

Roasted chicken breast
(4 ounces sliced breast from roasted chicken)
Soft polenta with Parmesan cheese
Eggplant, Zucchini, and Tomato Tian*
Double Chocolate Cake* with sliced strawberries

Calories	1,809
Protein	82.1 g
Carbohydrate	257.2 g
Fiber	48.7 g
Fat Total	57.8 g
Saturated	11.5 g
Mono	28.2 g
Poly	12.0 g
Cholesterol	100.2 mg
Arginine	4.1 g

DAY FIVE

BREAKFAST

Zucchini Frittata*
2 slices whole grain toast
1 tablespoon Apricot Spread*
1 cup soy or fat-free dairy yogurt

LUNCH

Red Pepper Gazpacho*
Mexican Tofu-Stuffed Pita*
Celery and Edamame Slaw*
1 wedge honeydew melon
¼ cup Soy Trail Mix*

DINNER

Moroccan Red Snapper*
1 cup couscous with chopped parsley and mint
1 cup Glazed Carrots*
1 cup blueberries

Calories	1,810
Protein	87.0 g
Carbohydrates	209.6 g
Fiber	36.8 g
Fat Total	77.8 g
Saturated	13.9 g
Mono	39.0 g
Poly	18.6 g
Cholesterol	127.2 mg
Arginine	4.0 g

DAY SIX

BREAKFAST

Pineapple Ginger Smoothie*
1 slice whole grain toast
1 tablespoon almond or soynut butter

LUNCH

Red Lentils with Beets and Tofu "Feta"*
8 Whole Wheat Pita Crisps*
½ cup diced cantaloupe

DINNER

Soy-Glazed Salmon*
Brown Rice Pilaf with Dill*
Endive and Watercress Salad with Hazelnuts*
Chocolate Raspberry Surprise*

Calories	1,889
Protein	88.2 g
Carbohydrates	221.6 g
Fiber	37.0 g
Fat Total	79.1 g
Saturated	17.5 g
Mono	36.8 g
Poly	19.0 g
Cholesterol	94.3 mg
Arginine	5.5 g

DAY SEVEN

BREAKFAST

1 cup orange juice
Banana Date-Nut Bread*

LUNCH

Quinoa with Broccoli, Sweet Potato, and Smoked Tofu*
Mesclun salad with edamame, sliced cucumber,
and Flax Vinaigrette*
1 cup fresh cherries or strawberries

DINNER

Chicken Wrap with Refried Beans*
Jicama, Edamame, and Red Pepper Salad*
1 cup diced watermelon

Calories	1,847
Protein	71.5 g
Carbohydrates	281.2 g
Fiber	31.2 g
Fat Total	61.7 g
Saturated	9.8 g
Mono	27.3 g
Poly	19.3 g
Cholesterol	72.1 mg
Arginine	4.6 g

DAY EIGHT

BREAKFAST

8 ounces orange juice
Tofu and Bacon Scrambler*
Bran Muffin*

LUNCH

1½ cups Green Pea Soup*
2 pumpernickel flatbread or whole grain crackers
Spinach and White Bean Salad*
1 nectarine or peach

DINNER

Roasted chicken breast
(4 ounces sliced breast from roasted chicken)
Braised Swiss Chard*
1 cup Bulgur Pilaf*
½ cup fruit sorbet

Calories	1,841
Protein	106.9 g
Carbohydrates	232.6 g
Fiber	44.9 g
Fat Total	66.0 g
Saturated	10.1 g
Mono	30.1 g
Poly	20.7 g
Cholesterol	114.4 mg
Arginine	6.2 g

DAY NINE

BREAKFAST

Creamy Oat Bran Porridge* with Flax Nut Topping*
2 tangerines

LUNCH

Salade Niçoise*
Whole Wheat Crostini* with 2 teaspoons Herb-Infused Olive Oil*
1 pear

DINNER

1 cup Chilled Beet Soup*
Grilled halibut, 5 ounces
Mango Mint Salsa*
Shelled edamame sautéed with olive oil and garlic
Double Chocolate Cake*

Calories	1,795
Protein	109.1 g
Carbohydrates	188.1 g
Fiber	31.3 g
Fat Total	78.6 g
Saturated	12.3 g
Mono	41.2 g
Poly	16.0 g
Cholesterol	100.5 mg
Arginine	3.9 g

DAY TEN

BREAKFAST

2 slices whole grain toast
2 tablespoons Apricot Spread*
2 tablespoons toasted sliced almonds
8 ounces soymilk or low-fat milk

LUNCH

2 cups Three Bean Soup*
Mesclun salad with Ginger Vinaigrette*
1 sliced Fuji or Jonagold apple
2 tablespoons soynut butter

DINNER

Tomato Bruschetta*
Linguini with Roasted Vegetable Sauce*
Braised Swiss Chard*
1 cup fresh berries

Calories	1,734
Protein	56.5 g
Carbohydrates	250.7 g
Fiber	58.1 g
Fat Total	67.7 g
Saturated	8.4 g
Mono	35.2 g
Poly	18.5 g
Cholesterol	3.0 mg
Arginine	2.8 g

DAY ELEVEN

BREAKFAST

1 cup orange juice
3 Blueberry Oat Pancakes*
½ cup fresh blueberries
3 tablespoons maple syrup

LUNCH

Smoked Salmon Roulades*
Crunchy Chopped Salad*
Sliced kiwi and strawberries

DINNER

Red Pepper Gazpacho*
Broiled salmon, 5 ounces
Brown Rice and Red Lentil Pilaf*
Sautéed spinach
1 cup raspberries

Calories	1,845
Protein	90.0 g
Carbohydrates	265.3 g
Fiber	35.7 g
Fat Total	52.6 g
Saturated	10.6 g
Mono	21.2 g
Poly	11.6 g
Cholesterol	200.0 mg
Arginine	4.1 g

DAY TWELVE

BREAKFAST

1 cup cubed fresh papaya
Hot Kashi cereal with Flax Nut Topping*
8 ounces soymilk or low-fat milk

LUNCH

Spinach and White Bean Salad*
1 sliced tomato
2 slices Swedish flatbread
2 cups diced cantaloupe
1 Soy'more*

DINNER

Roasted chicken breast
(4 ounces sliced breast from roasted chicken)
¾ cup Roasted Onions*
1 cup sautéed Brussels sprouts
Bulgur Pilaf*
Red Grape Macédoine*

Calories	1,833
Protein	82.8 g
Carbohydrates	266.9 g
Fiber	50.4 g
Fat Total	55.7 g
Saturated	9.0 g
Mono	22.1 g
Poly	13.6 g
Cholesterol	95.5 mg
Arginine	4.2 g

DAY THIRTEEN

BREAKFAST

Tropical Smoothie*
1 slice rye toast
1 tablespoon soy cream cheese

LUNCH

2 cups Butternut Squash, Chickpea, Tomato, and Corn Soup*
Spinach salad with Honey Mustard Dressing*
8 Whole Wheat Pita Crisps* with 2 teaspoons of
Herb-Infused Olive Oil*
Soy or fat-free dairy yogurt

DINNER

1 cup Chilled Beet Soup*
Soy-Glazed Salmon*
Glazed Carrots*
Wild Rice Salad*
1 cup fresh raspberries

Calories	1,815
Protein	80.9 g
Carbohydrates	225.5 g
Fiber	33.2 g
Fat Total	71.5 g
Saturated	14.1 g
Mono	33.6 g
Poly	17.9 g
Cholesterol	116.4 mg
Arginine	3.6 g

DAY FOURTEEN

BREAKFAST

1 cup fresh strawberries
1½ cups soy breakfast cereal with 1 tablespoon chopped walnuts
8 ounces soymilk or low-fat dairy milk

LUNCH

Turkey and Swiss Sandwich*
Romaine, watercress, and cherry tomato salad
with Honey Mustard Dressing*
1 cup Summer Fruit Salad*

DINNER

Broiled swordfish, 6 ounces
Stir-Fried Baby Bok Choy with Ginger*
Baked sweet potato
1 cup Cherry Berry Compote* with 1 cup vanilla soy frozen dessert

Calories	1,790
Protein	103.8 g
Carbohydrates	218.0 g
Fiber	40.8 g
Fat Total	63.8 g
Saturated	11.2 g
Mono	13.8 g
Poly	15.4 g
Cholesterol	122.8 mg
Arginine	5.8 g

The Recipes

BREAKFAST

APRICOT SPREAD
SERVES 8 (MAKES 1 CUP)

1 cup (6 ounces) dried apricots
3 strips orange zest, each 2 inches × 1 inch
¼ cup frozen apple juice concentrate
2 tablespoons honey
6 ounces (½ package) firm low-fat silken tofu (see p. 70 for
   information on types of tofu)
Juice of ½ lemon

1. Place the apricots, zest, juice concentrate, and honey in a medium saucepan. Add ½ cup water.
2. Bring just to a boil over medium-high heat. Cover tightly, reduce the heat, and simmer 20 minutes. The apricots should be puffed and soft when pierced with a knife.
3. Transfer the entire contents of the pot to a blender. Blend to a coarse puree, stopping often to scrape down the sides of the container. Add the tofu and lemon juice. Whirl to make a velvety, thick puree.
4. Scoop the spread into a container and cool to room temperature. Taste, adding a bit more lemon juice if it tastes "beany." This spread keeps, tightly covered, for up to 10 days in the refrigerator.

Nutrient Analysis: Apricot Spread (2 tablespoons)

Calories	97
Protein	2.2 g
Carbohydrates	22.1 g
Fiber	1.3 g
Fat Total	0.3 g
Saturated	0.0 g
Mono	0.0 g
Poly	0.1 g
Cholesterol	0.0 mg
Arginine	0.1 g

BANANA DATE-NUT BREAD
SERVES 9, MAKES 3 SMALL LOAVES

1 cup plus 2 teaspoons unbleached all-purpose flour
1 cup chopped pitted dates
½ cup whole wheat flour
1 teaspoon baking soda
½ teaspoon baking powder
¼ teaspoon salt
1 large egg
½ cup low-fat buttermilk
⅓ cup honey
3 tablespoons canola oil
1 teaspoon vanilla extract
1 medium banana, sliced
½ cup chopped walnuts

1. Place a rack in the center of the oven. Preheat the oven to 375°F. Spray three 5¾-inch × 3¼-inch × 2-inch metal or disposable foil loaf pans with cooking spray and set aside.
2. Place the 2 teaspoons of flour in a small bowl. Add the dates, tossing with your fingers to separate and coat them with the flour. Set aside.
3. In a large bowl, whisk to combine the remaining all-purpose flour, whole wheat flour, baking soda, baking powder, and salt.
4. In another bowl, lightly beat the egg. Add the buttermilk, honey, oil, and vanilla. Whisk to combine them. Pour this mixture all at once into the dry ingredients, whisking just to combine them, 9 or 10 strokes. Using a rubber spatula, mix in the dates, banana slices, and walnuts. Divide the batter among the three prepared pans, filling each about halfway. Set the pans on a baking sheet.
5. Bake 25 to 30 minutes, until the loaves are well browned and a straw inserted in the center comes out clean. Let the cakes cool in the pan for 10 minutes. Turn them out and cool the cakes completely on a rack. Wrap in aluminum foil. The loaves will be moister and taste better the next day. The loaves keep, unrefrigerated, for 5 days. Individual loaves can be wrapped in plastic, then foil, and frozen. Defrost frozen loaves in the refrigerator.

Nutrient Analysis: Banana Date-Nut Bread (One-third loaf)

Calories	253
Protein	4.2 g
Carbohydrates	40.8 g
Fiber	2.8 g
Fat Total	9.6 g
Saturated	1.0 g
Mono	3.5 g
Poly	4.5 g
Cholesterol	24.4 mg
Arginine	0.2 g

BLUEBERRY OAT PANCAKES

SERVES 6 (MAKES 12)

1 cup rolled oats (not quick-cooking or instant)
1 cup low-fat or fat-free buttermilk
1 extra-large egg
1 tablespoon sugar
Pinch of salt
2 tablespoons plus 2 teaspoons canola oil
1 cup blueberries
6 ounces (½ package) firm silken tofu, finely chopped (see note)
½ cup unbleached all-purpose flour
¼ teaspoon baking powder
¼ teaspoon baking soda
Maple syrup or blueberry syrup, as accompaniment (optional)

1. In a medium bowl, combine the oats and buttermilk. Set aside for 20 to 30 minutes.
2. In a small bowl, whisk together the egg, sugar, salt, and 2 tablespoons of the oil. Blend this mixture into the oats. Mix in the blueberries and tofu. Add the flour, baking powder, and baking soda, mixing to combine them.
3. Heat a griddle or heavy, large skillet over medium-high heat. Grease lightly, using 1 teaspoon of the oil and wiping out the excess with a paper towel. Drop the batter by scant quarter cups into the hot pan, flattening it slightly, to make 4-inch pancakes. Space the pancakes about 2 inches apart. Cook until well browned, 2 to 3 minutes. Turn, reduce the heat to medium-low, and cook until

the pancakes feel firm in the center when pressed with a finger-tip, about 2 minutes. Transfer to a plate. Serve as the pancakes are done. Repeat, using up the remaining batter. Pass maple syrup or warm blueberry syrup, if desired.

NOTE: Use the tofu sold in boxes, such as Mori-Nu, in firm texture. If desired, use the reduced-fat kind. (See p. 70 for information on types of tofu.)

Nutrient Analysis: Blueberry Oat Pancakes (2 pancakes, not including maple or blueberry syrup)

Calories	205
Protein	7.8 g
Carbohydrates	24.2 g
Fiber	2.3 g
Fat Total	8.7 g
Saturated	1.2 g
Mono	4.4 g
Poly	2.4 g
Cholesterol	43.5 mg
Arginine	0.1 g

BRAN MUFFINS
MAKES 12

¼ cup soy flour
1 cup wheat bran
⅓ cup boiling water
1 cup all-purpose flour
1 teaspoon baking soda
1 teaspoon ground cinnamon
⅛ teaspoon ground nutmeg
½ teaspoon salt
½ cup dehydrated sugar cane juice (Sucanat)
¼ cup canola oil
1 large egg
1 cup low-fat or fat-free buttermilk
6 chopped black mission figs
6 whole dried apricots, chopped
1 tablespoon sesame seeds

1. Preheat the oven to 325°F. Spread the soy flour in a pie plate or other shallow baking pan. Roast it, stirring every 2 minutes, until it is the color of butterscotch pudding, about 10 minutes. Set aside to cool. This step can be done several days ahead. You can also toast several cups of flour at a time, storing the unused portion in a tightly covered jar.

2. Increase the temperature to 350°F. Toast the bran, using the same method as above, until it is the color of whole wheat bread, about 8 minutes. Set aside to cool. This can be done up to 1 day ahead.

3. Preheat the oven to 400°F. Place paper muffin cups in the cavities of a 12-muffin tin. Place the bran in a small bowl. Pour in the boiling water. Stir until the bran is completely moistened, then set aside.

4. Combine the soy flour, flour, baking soda, cinnamon, nutmeg, and salt in a small bowl. In a medium bowl, using a wooden spoon, work the dehydrated sugar cane juice and oil together until completely moistened and grainy looking. Beat in the egg until well blended. Add ⅓ of the buttermilk and stir. Add ⅓ of the dry ingredients, stirring just until they are blended. Do not worry if there are some lumps. Repeat twice more with the remaining buttermilk and dry ingredients. Work the batter against the side of the bowl with the back of the spoon to remove some of the lumps, allowing smaller ones to remain.

5. Mix the dried fruit into the batter. Mix in the bran. Spoon the batter into the prepared muffin tin, filling the cups almost to the top. Sprinkle ¼ teaspoon sesame seeds over each muffin.

6. Bake 20 minutes, until a bamboo skewer inserted into the middle of a muffin comes out clean. Cool 5 minutes in the pan. Using tongs, transfer the muffins to a rack. Cool completely. These muffins keep about 4 days, stored in a plastic bag.

Nutrient Analysis: Bran Muffins (1 muffin)

Calories	162
Protein	4.6 g
Carbohydrates	22.1 g
Fiber	4.3 g
Fat Total	6.6 g
Saturated	0.8 g
Mono	3.2 g
Poly	2.3 g
Cholesterol	18.9 mg
Arginine	0.1 g

MUESLI

SERVES 4

1 cup rolled oats (not quick-cooking or instant)
½ cup oat bran
¼ cup toasted wheat germ
3 whole dried apricots, chopped
3 tablespoons dried sweet cherries, coarsely chopped
¼ cup (¾ ounce) sliced almonds

½ small Fuji apple, with skin, shredded
6 ounces soymilk

1. In a large bowl, combine the oats, bran, wheat germ, apricots, and cherries.
2. In a heavy, dry skillet over medium-high heat, toast the almonds, stirring constantly, until they start turning golden. Add to the muesli mixture.
3. To serve, combine ½ cup muesli, the shredded apple, and soymilk. Cover and refrigerate at least 2 hours, up to overnight.

Nutrient Analysis: Muesli (1 serving)

Calories	294
Protein	13.7 g
Carbohydrates	46.5 g
Fiber	11.0 g
Fat Total	9.1 g
Saturated	1.1 g
Mono	3.2 g
Poly	3.4 g
Cholesterol	0.0 mg
Arginine	1.0 g

CREAMY OAT BRAN PORRIDGE
SERVES 2

1 cup unsweetened soymilk
½ cup oat bran
3 tablespoons dried currants
Pinch of salt
⅛ teaspoon ground cinnamon
2 tablespoons Flax Nut Topping (see below)

1. Pour the soymilk into a medium saucepan. Add 1 cup water. Stir in the oat bran. Add the currants and salt. Set the pan over medium-high heat.
2. Cook, stirring occasionally, until the liquid begins to boil. Reduce the heat to medium and cook, stirring often, until the porridge is thick and creamy, about 10 minutes. Divide the porridge between two bowls. Sprinkle each with half the cinnamon and a tablespoon of Flax Nut Topping. Serve immediately.

Nutrient Analysis: Creamy Oat Bran Porridge (1 serving, including Flax Nut Topping)

Calories	233
Protein	10.9 g
Carbohydrates	34.7 g
Fiber	5.9 g
Fat Total	10.1 g
Saturated	1.2 g
Mono	4.7 g
Poly	3.8 g
Cholesterol	0.0 mg
Arginine	0.5 g

FLAX NUT TOPPING
SERVES 8 (MAKES 1 CUP)

½ cup slivered almonds, coarsely chopped
½ cup peeled hazelnuts, coarsely chopped
3 tablespoons flaxseeds (see note)

1. Place a rack in the center of the oven. Preheat the oven to 350°F.
2. Spread the nuts in one layer in a shallow baking dish. Roast until they are lightly browned, about 10 minutes, shaking the pan every 2 or 3 minutes so the nuts color evenly. Place the nuts in a bowl to cool.
3. Grind the flaxseeds in a clean coffee grinder or spice mill until they are a coarse meal. Add them to the nuts. Flax Nut Topping keeps a week or more in a tightly sealed jar in the refrigerator.

NOTE: Flaxseeds are sold at natural and health food stores.

Nutrient Analysis: Flax Nut Topping (1 tablespoon)

Calories	114
Protein	3.5 g
Carbohydrates	4.1 g
Fiber	2.5 g
Fat Total	9.9 g
Saturated	0.7 g
Mono	6.3 g
Poly	2.3 g
Cholesterol	0.0 mg
Arginine	0.4 g

PINEAPPLE GINGER SMOOTHIE
SERVES 1

1 cup diced ripe pineapple, frozen if desired
¾-inch piece gingerroot, peeled and chopped
2 teaspoons flaxseeds
½ cup orange juice
6 mint leaves
1 cup plain or vanilla soymilk

1. In a blender, puree the pineapple with the ginger, flaxseeds, orange juice, and mint. Add the soymilk and whirl to blend. Serve immediately.

Nutrient Analysis: Pineapple Ginger Smoothie

Calories	249
Protein	9.6 g

Carbohydrates	40.2 g
Fiber	7.2 g
Fat Total	7.7 g
Saturated	0.8 g
Mono	1.3 g
Poly	3.7 g
Cholesterol	0.0 mg
Arginine	0.6 g

PUMPKIN MUFFINS

SERVES 12

Topping

2 tablespoons rolled oats (not quick-cooking or instant)
1 tablespoon unroasted pumpkin seeds
1 tablespoon whole salted soynuts
1 tablespoon unroasted sunflower seeds
2 teaspoons unhulled sesame seeds
1 tablespoon brown sugar

Muffins

1½ cups unbleached all-purpose flour
½ cup stone-ground whole wheat flour
1½ teaspoons baking powder
1 teaspoon baking soda
1 teaspoon ground cinnamon
½ teaspoon ground ginger (optional)
1 teaspoon salt
1 large egg
1 large egg white
1 lightly packed cup brown sugar
1 cup canned pureed pumpkin
¼ cup canola oil
¾ cup golden raisins
¾ cup chopped walnuts

1. Place a rack in the center of the oven. Preheat the oven to 375°F. Spray a 12-cavity muffin pan with cooking spray and set aside.

2. Combine the oats, pumpkin seeds, soynuts, sunflower seeds, sesame seeds, and brown sugar for the topping in a small bowl and set aside.

3. In a medium bowl, combine the flour, whole wheat flour, baking powder, baking soda, cinnamon, ginger (if using), and salt. In a large bowl, whisk the eggs. With a wooden spoon, mix the sugar into the eggs until no lumps remain. Stir in the pumpkin, then the oil, raisins, and walnuts.

4. Add the dry ingredients to the wet mixture. Mix just until they are combined; do not overmix. Spoon the mixture into the prepared pan, filling the pan cavities almost to the top.

5. Bake 20 minutes, or until a bamboo skewer inserted into the center comes out clean. Turn onto a rack to cool completely before serving. These muffins keep 2 days wrapped in foil. Wrapped individually, the muffins freeze well. Let sit at room temperature to defrost.

Nutrient Analysis: Pumpkin Muffins (1 muffin)

Calories (1 muffin)	277
Protein	6.3 g
Carbohydrates	39.6 g
Fiber	2.9 g
Fat Total	11.0 g
Saturated	0.9 g
Mono	4.2 g
Poly	4.7 g
Cholesterol	17.7 mg
Arginine	0.4 g

TOFU AND BACON SCRAMBLER
SERVES 2

14 to 16 ounce package firm tofu, drained (see note)
1½ teaspoons canola oil
1 small onion, finely chopped
½ medium green bell pepper, finely chopped
4 medium white mushrooms, stemmed and thinly sliced
⅛ teaspoon ground turmeric
¼ teaspoon soy sauce

Pinch of cayenne pepper
2 strips Morningstar Farms Breakfast Strips or Worthington
Stripples, cooked according to package directions and
crumbled
Salt and freshly ground black pepper

1. Cut the tofu into 8 pieces. One at a time, place each piece of the tofu in the palm of one hand. Cup the other hand over it, as if you are applauding. Holding the tofu over the sink, gently press your hands together until half the moisture has been squeezed out of the tofu. It should be somewhat crushed and resemble broken-up custard. Place the tofu in a small bowl. Repeat, pressing all the tofu.

2. In a medium nonstick skillet, heat the oil over medium-high heat. Sauté the onion until it is browned, about 5 minutes. Add the green pepper, cooking until it is bright green, about 1 minute. Add the mushrooms. Cook, stirring occasionally, until they give up their liquid. Continue cooking until they are lightly browned.

3. Add the tofu. Immediately add the turmeric, soy sauce, and cayenne, stirring with a wooden spoon until the tofu is lightly colored and looks moist. Mix in the crumbled bacon. Season to taste with salt and pepper. Serve immediately.

NOTE: The firm tofu from Nasoya, Hinoichi, or Azumaya produces a scrambler resembling soft eggs. Using extra-firm tofu, it is more like well-cooked eggs. If the brand of tofu used is grainy or too hard, or if reduced-fat tofu is used, the scrambler will be dry and pasty tasting. Boxed tofu, such as Mori-Nu, will be very moist and taste mushy, no matter the texture used.

Nutrient Analysis: Tofu and Bacon Scrambler (1 serving)

Calories	339
Protein	28.4 g
Carbohydrates	18.2 g
Fiber	6.2 g
Fat Total	19.9 g
Saturated	2.6 g
Mono	5.6 g
Poly	10.3 g
Cholesterol	0.2 mg
Arginine	1.7 g

TROPICAL SMOOTHIE

SERVES 1

½ *medium banana, sliced*
½ *medium ripe mango (about 1 cup flesh)*
4 frozen strawberries
½ *cup low-fat or fat-free buttermilk*
½ *cup orange juice*
2 ice cubes

1. Place the banana, mango, and strawberries in a blender. Add the buttermilk, juice, and ice. Whirl until well blended and smooth. Serve in a tall glass.

Nutrient Analysis: Tropical Smoothie

Calories	242
Protein	26.2 g
Carbohydrates	54.0 g
Fiber	4.4 g
Fat Total	1.9 g
Saturated	0.9 g
Mono	0.5 g
Poly	0.2 g
Cholesterol	4.3 mg
Arginine	0.3 g

ZUCCHINI FRITTATA

SERVES 4

1 tablespoon extra virgin olive oil
1 large zucchini (about 10 ounces), cut in ¼-inch slices
½ *teaspoon salt, or to taste, and freshly ground pepper*
1 scallion, green part only, thinly sliced
3 large egg whites
1 large egg
1 tablespoon grated Parmesan cheese

1. Heat the oil in a medium nonstick skillet over medium-high heat. Add the zucchini; the pan will be very crowded. Cook 4 minutes.

Sprinkle with half the salt. Add the scallions. Cook until the zucchini softens and just covers the bottom of the pan, about 3 minutes.

2. Meanwhile, beat the egg whites, egg, cheese, and remaining salt in a bowl until they are well blended.

3. Pour the egg mixture over the squash. As the eggs set at the edge of the pan, keep lifting them with a fork, tilting the pan so the liquid eggs can run to the outer edge. Cook, reducing the heat to medium, until the eggs are well set and the frittata is browned on the bottom, about 6 minutes.

4. Remove the pan from the heat. Shake it so the frittata slides easily. Invert a plate and set it over the pan. Holding the plate firmly in place, invert, so the frittata falls onto it. Slide the frittata back into the pan. Replace it over the heat. Cook until the frittata is lightly browned on the bottom, about 3 minutes. Slide the frittata onto a clean plate. Spinkle with the remaining ¼ teaspoon salt and freshly ground black pepper to taste. Cut in quarters and serve. Or let the frittata cool and serve at room temperature.

Nutrient Analysis: Zucchini Frittata (1 serving)

Calories	82
Protein	5.7 g
Carbohydrates	2.8 g
Fiber	1.0 g
Fat Total	5.4 g
Saturated	1.2 g
Mono	3.3 g
Poly	0.6 g
Cholesterol	54.2 mg
Arginine	0.3 g

SOUPS

BLACK BEAN SOUP
SERVES 4

1 tablespoon canola oil
1 medium onion, chopped
1 large shallot, chopped
1 small green bell pepper, chopped
1 small red bell pepper, chopped
2 portobello mushrooms, stemmed and chopped
3 large tomatoes, seeded and chopped
2 15-ounce cans black beans, rinsed and drained
1 teaspoon dried oregano
1 teaspoon dried thyme
1 bay leaf
Salt and freshly ground black pepper

1. Heat the oil in a large Dutch oven or heavy saucepan over medium-high heat. Sauté the onion, shallot, and green and red peppers until the onion is translucent, about 4 minutes. Add the mushrooms. Cook, stirring occasionally, until they give up their liquid, about 4 minutes. Stir in the tomatoes and cook until they soften, about 2 minutes.
2. Add the drained beans. Pour in 3 cups water. Add the oregano, thyme, and bay leaf. Bring the soup to a boil, reduce the heat, and simmer, uncovered, until the vegetables are very soft, about 20 minutes. Let the soup sit to cool slightly.
3. Remove the bay leaf. Puree the soup, in two batches, if necessary. Make it smooth or leave it slightly pulpy, as you prefer. Season the soup to taste with salt and pepper. Serve hot.

Nutrient Analysis: Black Bean Soup (1 serving)

Calories	231
Protein	11.5 g
Carbohydrates	45.9 g
Fiber	14.6 g
Fat Total	4.1 g
Saturated	0.3 g
Mono	2.1 g
Poly	1.2 g
Cholesterol	0.0 mg
Arginine	0.9 g

CHILLED BEET SOUP

SERVES 4

2 medium beets
1 cup buttermilk (see note)
¼ cup plain yogurt (see note)
1 tablespoon fresh lemon juice
Salt and freshly ground black pepper
¼ cup chopped fresh dill
2 tablespoons snipped chives

1. Tear off the tops of the beets, leaving on about 2 inches of stems. Scrub the beets well. Place them in a deep pot. Add 3 cups cold water. Cook over high heat until the water boils. Reduce the heat, cover, and cook until the beets are soft when a sharp knife is inserted in the center, about 40 minutes. Cool the beets in their cooking liquid. Measure off ½ cup of the cooking liquid and discard the rest.

2. Cut away the top and bottom of the beets. Using your fingers, slip off the peel. Coarsely chop the beets. Place them in blender. Pour in the reserved cooking liquid, the buttermilk, yogurt, and lemon juice. Puree until the soup is smooth. Season it to taste with salt and pepper.

3. Chill the soup completely, at least 2 hours. Before serving, check the seasoning, adding more lemon juice, salt, and pepper, if needed. Divide the soup among 4 shallow bowls. Garnish each serving with a quarter of the dill and chives. This soup keeps in the refrigerator, tightly covered, for 3 days.

NOTE: Use regular, low-fat or fat-free buttermilk. Use regular or low-fat, but not fat-free, yogurt.

Nutrient Analysis: Chilled Beet Soup (1 serving, including 1% buttermilk and low-fat yogurt)

Calories	57
Protein	3.9 g
Carbohydrates	8.5 g
Fiber	0.4 g
Fat Total	1.2 g
Saturated	0.7 g
Mono	0.3 g
Poly	0.0 g
Cholesterol	5.7 mg
Arginine	0.0 g

GREEN PEA SOUP

SERVES 4

2 tablespoons canola oil
1 small carrot, chopped
1 medium celery rib, chopped
1 medium leek, white part only, chopped
1 medium onion, chopped
1 cup dried split green peas
4 cups defatted, low-sodium chicken broth, or vegetable broth
1 garlic clove, chopped
6 parsley sprigs
½ teaspoon dried thyme
1 bay leaf
Salt and freshly ground black pepper

1. Heat the oil in a deep, heavy saucepan over medium-high heat. Sauté the carrot, celery, leek, and onion until the onion is translucent, about 4 minutes. Cover tightly, reduce the heat to medium, and cook until the vegetables release their juices, 5 minutes.
2. Add the peas, broth, garlic, parsley, thyme, and bay leaf. Bring to a boil, reduce the heat, and cook the soup, covered, until the peas are falling apart, about 45 minutes.
3. Remove the bay leaf and parsley sprigs. Let the soup sit for 20 minutes to cool slightly. Puree in a blender, in two batches, if necessary. Season to taste with salt and pepper. This soup keeps, tightly covered in the refrigerator, for up to 4 days.

Nutrient Analysis: Green Pea Soup (1 serving)

Calories	299
Protein	18.0 g
Carbohydrates	37.0 g
Fiber	14.0 g
Fat Total	8.9 g
Saturated	1.0 g
Mono	4.7 g
Poly	2.6 g
Cholesterol	0.0 mg
Arginine	1.2 g

BUTTERNUT SQUASH, CHICKPEA, TOMATO, AND CORN SOUP

SERVES 4

1 tablespoon canola oil
1 large garlic clove, minced
1 medium onion, chopped
2 cups ½-inch cubes peeled butternut squash
½ green bell pepper, chopped
1 teaspoon salt
1 teaspoon ground cumin
1 teaspoon paprika
½ teaspoon dried basil
3 cups defatted, low-sodium chicken broth
1 bay leaf
1 large tomato, seeded and chopped
1 14½-ounce can chickpeas, drained
1 cup frozen corn kernels
Freshly ground black pepper

1. In a large saucepan or small Dutch oven, heat the oil over medium-high heat. Mix in the garlic, onion, squash, green pepper, and salt. Sauté until the onion is translucent and starts to soften, 5 minutes, stirring occasionally.

2. Mix in the cumin and paprika, stirring until they smell fragrant. Add the basil, broth, and bay leaf. Bring to a boil, cover, reduce the heat, and simmer 10 minutes. Add the tomato, chickpeas, and corn. Simmer, uncovered, 10 minutes. Remove the bay leaf. Season to taste with pepper. Tightly covered, this soup keeps up to 4 days in the refrigerator, and it freezes well.

Nutrient Analysis: Butternut Squash, Chickpea, Tomato, and Corn Soup (1 serving)

Calories	150
Protein	5.3 g
Carbohydrates	24.3 g
Fiber	5.1 g
Fat Total	5.3 g
Saturated	0.9 g
Mono	2.1 g
Poly	1.3 g

| Cholesterol | 2.9 mg |
| Arginine | 0.2 g |

RED PEPPER GAZPACHO
SERVES 4

1 large red bell pepper, roasted, seeded, and diced
2 large cloves garlic
1½ cups tomato juice
1 slice stale multigrain bread, crusts removed (see note)
1 tablespoon white wine vinegar
1 teaspoon extra virgin olive oil
3 generous dashes hot pepper sauce
Freshly ground black pepper
⅔ cup finely diced cucumber
⅔ cup finely diced green bell pepper
⅔ cup finely diced tomato
⅔ cup finely diced raw zucchini
⅔ cup finely diced celery (optional)
⅔ cup finely diced red onion (optional)

1. In a blender, combine the red pepper and garlic. Add ½ cup of the tomato juice. Puree to a coarse pulp. Add the remaining tomato juice and whirl to blend.
2. Break the stale bread into 4 pieces. Puree them into the soup, which should be slightly pulpy at this point.
3. Blend in the vinegar, oil, hot pepper sauce, and ground pepper to taste. Transfer the soup to a container, cover, and chill 3 to 4 hours or overnight.
4. Pour the chilled soup into individual bowls. Add a scant tablespoon of the diced cucumber, green pepper, tomato, and zucchini, plus the celery and onion, if using.

NOTE: If the bread is not stale, dry it out in a 350°F oven for about 8 minutes, turning it once. Cool and trim away the crust before using.

Calories	67
Protein	2.3 g
Carbohydrates	13.2 g
Fiber	3.1 g
Fat Total	1.6 g
Saturated	0.2 g
Mono	0.9 g
Poly	0.2 g
Cholesterol	0.0 mg
Arginine	0.1 g

THREE BEAN SOUP

SERVES 8

2 tablespoons extra virgin olive oil
1 medium onion, chopped
1 small carrot, finely chopped
½ cup chopped fennel
1 ounce prosciutto ham, finely chopped (optional)
¼ cup pearl barley
¼ cup chopped flatleaf parsley
1 15-ounce can chickpeas
1 15-ounce can kidney beans, rinsed and drained
1 15-ounce can white or navy beans, rinsed and drained
1 large yellow-fleshed potato, peeled and cut in ½-inch pieces
2 tablespoons tomato paste
1 teaspoon dried sage
1 bay leaf
Salt and freshly ground black pepper
Grated Parmesan cheese (optional)

1. Heat the oil in a small Dutch oven or heavy, large saucepan over medium-high heat. Sauté the onion, carrot, fennel, and prosciutto, if using, until the onion is translucent and soft, 5 minutes.
2. Add the barley and parsley. Pour in 4 cups water. Bring to a boil, reduce the heat, and simmer, uncovered, for 20 minutes.
3. Add the chickpeas, with their liquid, the drained kidney and white beans, and the potato. Stir in the tomato paste and sage. Add the

bay leaf. Season to taste with salt and pepper. Simmer until the barley is soft and the potatoes are cooked, about 20 minutes. Remove the bay leaf. Serve, accompanied by grated Parmesan, if desired. This soup keeps, tightly covered in the refrigerator, for 5 days.

Nutrient Analysis: Three Bean Soup (1 serving, not including Parmesan cheese)

Calories	217
Protein	10.3 g
Carbohydrates	35.7 g
Fiber	9.7 g
Fat Total	5.4 g
Saturated	0.6 g
Mono	3.2 g
Poly	1.0 g
Cholesterol	2.5 mg
Arginine	0.4 g

SALADS AND DRESSINGS

CELERY AND EDAMAME SLAW
SERVES 4

1 cup frozen shelled edamame
4 medium ribs celery
¼ medium red bell pepper, finely chopped
2 tablespoons finely chopped red onion
¼ cup chopped flatleaf parsley, lightly packed
1 tablespoon chopped celery leaves
Juice of ½ lime
1 teaspoon salt
1 tablespoon canola oil
Freshly ground black pepper

1. Cook the edamame in salted boiling water for 3 minutes. Drain and place in a medium bowl.
2. Cut the celery ribs diagonally, at a 45-degree angle, into ⅛-inch

slices. Add to the edamame. Add the red pepper, onion, parsley, celery leaves, lime juice, salt, and oil. Using a fork, toss to combine. Season to taste with pepper. Cover with plastic wrap and refrigerate 30 minutes. Adjust seasoning to taste and serve. This salad keeps for 1 day, tightly covered in the refrigerator.

Nutrient Analysis: Celery and Edamame Slaw (1 serving)

Calories	43
Protein	0.5 g
Carbohydrates	2.9 g
Fiber	1.0 g
Fat Total	3.5 g
Saturated	0.3 g
Mono	2.0 g
Poly	1.0 g
Cholesterol	0.0 mg
Arginine	0.7 g

CRUNCHY CHOPPED SALAD

SERVES 2

3 medium radishes, chopped
1 small green bell pepper
1 large or 2 medium scallions, green and white parts, chopped
½ medium cucumber, peeled, seeded, and diced
1 tablespoon soy sour cream
1 tablespoon fresh lemon juice
2 tablespoons chopped fresh dill
Salt and freshly ground black pepper
1 bunch arugula

1. Place the radishes, bell pepper, scallions, cucumber, sour cream, and lemon juice in a medium bowl, and stir to combine. Add the dill. Using a fork, stir to combine. Season to taste with salt and pepper.
2. Cut the stems from the arugula. Stack the leaves. Cut the arugula crosswise into ¾-inch strips. Arrange half the greens to make a bed

on each of two salad plates. Heap half the chopped salad on each plate. Serve immediately.

Nutrient Analysis: Crunchy Chopped Salad (1 serving)

Calories	47
Protein	1.4 g
Carbohydrate	7.3 g
Fiber	2.2 g
Fat Total	1.7 g
Saturated	1.3 g
Mono	0.1 g
Poly	0.1 g
Cholesterol	0.0 mg
Arginine	0.0 g

ENDIVE AND WATERCRESS SALAD WITH HAZELNUTS

SERVES 4

¼ cup hazelnuts
1 large bunch watercress
1 large endive
2 tablespoons Honey Mustard Dressing (p. 125)

1. Preheat the oven to 350°F.
2. Place the nuts in a shallow baking dish or pie plate. Roast them until their skins crack and the nuts are lightly colored, 10 to 12 minutes, shaking the pan every 2 to 3 minutes so the nuts color evenly. Spread them onto a dishtowel. Rub vigorously to remove as much skin from the nuts as possible. Set the nuts aside to cool. This can be done up to 2 days ahead, with the roasted nuts stored in an airtight container.
3. Tear off the tender sprigs of watercress, discarding the tough stems. There should be about 4 cups. Place in a bowl. Cut the endive crosswise into ½-inch slices. Add to the cress, pulling the slices apart.
4. Add the dressing and toss to coat. Divide the salad among 4 plates. Coarsely chop the nuts. Sprinkle them over the salad and serve.

Nutrient Analysis: Endive and Watercress Salad with Hazelnuts (1 serving)

Calories	88
Protein	2.2 g
Carbohydrate	3.7 g
Fiber	1.7 g
Fat Total	7.9 g
Saturated	0.7 g
Mono	5.7 g
Poly	1.1 g
Cholesterol	0.0 mg
Arginine	0.2 g

JICAMA, EDAMAME, AND RED PEPPER SALAD
SERVES 4

½ medium jicama, peeled
1 small red pepper, seeded
1 cup cooked shelled edamame
1 large or 2 medium scallions, green part only, thinly sliced
Juice of 1 orange
1 tablespoon fresh lime juice
¼ teaspoon ground cumin
Pinch of cayenne pepper
Salt and freshly ground black pepper

1. Place the jicama cut-side down on a cutting board. Cut it vertically into ½-inch slices. Stack 2 slices. Cut the slices lengthwise into ½-inch strips. Cut the strips crosswise into 1-inch batons. Place the cut jicama in a medium bowl. Repeat, cutting up all the jicama.
2. Cut the red pepper vertically into ¼-inch strips. Add the red pepper to the jicama. Add the edamame and scallions.
3. In a small bowl, whisk the orange juice, lime juice, cumin, and cayenne together. Season the dressing to taste with salt and pepper. Pour it over the vegetables, tossing with a fork to blend. Serve immediately or cover and refrigerate. This salad is best served the day it is made, but it will keep, tightly covered in the refrigerator, for up to 24 hours.

Nutrient Analysis: Jicama, Edamame, and Red Pepper
Salad (1 serving)

Calories	111
Protein	6.6 g
Carbohydrates	16.0 g
Fiber	6.6 g
Fat Total	3.1 g
Saturated	0.4 g
Mono	0.6 g
Poly	1.4 g
Cholesterol	0.0 mg
Arginine	0.5 g

ROMAINE SALAD WITH
SHAVED PARMIGIANO-REGGIANO

SERVES 1

10 inner leaves romaine lettuce
1 tablespoon fresh lemon juice
¼ teaspoon salt
2 teaspoons extra virgin olive oil
Freshly ground black pepper
4 or 5 long curls (½ ounce) Parmigiano-Reggiano cheese

1. Tear the lettuce into 4-inch pieces. Leave the smallest leaves whole. Place in salad bowl.
2. Whisk together the lemon juice and salt. Whisk in the oil. Season to taste with the pepper. Pour the dressing over the greens. Toss to coat the lettuce.
3. Holding a chunk of Parmigiano-Reggiano over the greens, use a vegetable peeler to shave four or five long curls from the cheese into the salad and serve.

Nutrient Analysis: Romaine Salad with Shaved Parmigiano-
Reggiano

Calories	158
Protein	6.8 g
Carbohydrates	4.3 g
Fiber	1.8 g

Fat Total	13.2 g
Saturated	3.7 g
Mono	8.3 g
Poly	1.0 g
Cholesterol	9.6 mg
Arginine	0.3 g

SPINACH AND WHITE BEAN SALAD

SERVES 4

4 lightly packed cups baby spinach leaves
1 cup canned cannellini or white beans
1 small orange bell pepper
½ medium Hass avocado, cubed
¼ cup thinly sliced sweet onion, in crescents
1 cup canned mandarin orange sections
¼ cup fresh orange juice
2 tablespoons fresh lemon juice
1 tablespoon rice vinegar
Salt and freshly ground black pepper
2 teaspoons extra virgin olive oil

1. For the salad, wash and dry the spinach. Place the leaves in a large salad bowl. Rinse and drain the beans. Add them to the spinach. Cut the pepper vertically into quarters. Cut away the seeds and ribs. Cut each piece crosswise into ½-inch slices. Arrange the pepper slices over the beans and spinach. Add the avocado, onion, and orange sections.
2. For the dressing, in a small bowl, combine the orange and lemon juice with the vinegar. Whisk in salt and pepper to taste. Whisk in the oil.
3. To serve, pour the dressing over the salad. Toss immediately or present it at the table and toss. Serve at once.

Nutrient Analysis: Spinach and White Bean Salad
(1 serving)

Calories	166
Protein	5.3 g
Carbohydrates	26.4 g

Fiber	5.4 g
Fat Total	6.5 g
Saturated	0.9 g
Mono	4.2 g
Poly	0.7 g
Cholesterol	0.0 mg
Arginine	0.3 g

TUNA, APPLE, AND ARUGULA SALAD

SERVES 2

4 red lettuce leaves
1 small bunch arugula, stemmed, rinsed, and dried
1 6-ounce can water-packed albacore tuna, drained
1 Gala or Crispin apple, cored and thinly sliced
1 medium green bell pepper, seeded and cut into thin strips
2 tablespoons fresh lemon juice
½ teaspoon salt, or to taste
Freshly ground black pepper
2 tablespoons extra virgin olive oil

1. Tear the lettuce and arugula into bite-size pieces. Arrange the greens in a salad bowl. Heap the tuna in the center, on top of the greens. Arrange the apple slices in a ring around the tuna. Arrange the green pepper on top of the apple.
2. In a small bowl, whisk together the lemon juice, salt, pepper, and olive oil. Pour the dressing over the salad and toss. Divide the salad between two plates and serve.

NOTE: If the apple slices are tossed with 1 teaspoon lemon juice, this salad can be made up to 3 hours ahead. Cover tightly with plastic wrap and refrigerate. Add dressing and toss just before serving.

Nutrient Analysis: Tuna, Apple, and Arugula Salad (1 serving)

Calories	320
Protein	23.2 g
Carbohydrates	20.1 g
Fiber	5.4 g

Fat Total	17.3 g
Saturated	2.7 g
Mono	11.5 g
Poly	2.6 g
Cholesterol	35.7 mg
Arginine	1.3 g

WILD RICE SALAD

SERVES 6

1 15-ounce can *chickpeas, rinsed and drained*
2 tablespoons extra virgin olive oil
3 cups cooked wild rice
1 medium green bell pepper, seeded and finely chopped
1 small red bell pepper, seeded and finely chopped
1 small red onion, finely chopped
½ cup chopped flatleaf parsley
2 tablespoons fresh lemon juice
Salt and freshly ground black pepper

1. Preheat the oven to 400°F.
2. In a shallow heatproof dish, toss the chickpeas with one tablespoon of the oil. Bake until they are lightly colored, 15 to 20 minutes, stirring the beans twice so they roast evenly. Transfer the chickpeas to a large bowl.
3. Add the rice, green and red peppers, onion, parsley, lemon juice, and remaining tablespoon of oil to the bowl. Toss with a fork. Season the salad to taste with salt and pepper. This salad keeps, tightly covered in the refrigerator, for up to 4 days.

Nutrient Analysis: Wild Rice Salad (1 serving)

Calories	221
Protein	7.2 g
Carbohydrates	36.4 g
Fiber	5.4 g
Fat Total	5.9 g
Saturated	0.8 g
Mono	3.8 g
Poly	1.0 g

Cholesterol	0.0 mg
Arginine	0.6 g

FLAX VINAIGRETTE

MAKES ½ CUP

1 small garlic clove, halved
¼ cup white or red wine vinegar
1 tablespoon fresh lemon juice
2 teaspoons Dijon-style mustard
½ teaspoon salt
2 tablespoons extra virgin olive oil
2 tablespoons flaxseed oil (see note)
Freshly ground black pepper

1. Combine the garlic, vinegar, lemon juice, mustard, salt, and oils in a jar. Shake to combine. Season to taste with pepper. This dressing keeps, tightly covered in the refrigerator, for up to 3 days.

N O T E : Flaxseed oil is sold at natural and health food stores, often in the refrigerator section.

Nutrient Analysis: Flax Vinaigrette (1 tablespoon)

Calories	64
Protein	0.1 g
Carbohydrates	1.0 g
Fiber	0.0 g
Fat Total	7.0 g
Saturated	0.8 g
Mono	3.3 g
Poly	2.7 g
Cholesterol	0.0 mg
Arginine	0.0 g

GINGER VINAIGRETTE

MAKES ½ CUP

2 tablespoons grated ginger
1 tablespoon finely chopped shallots
¼ cup rice vinegar
1 tablespoon fresh lemon juice
1 teaspoon red wine or ½ teaspoon soy sauce
½ teaspoon salt
¼ cup canola oil
Freshly ground black pepper

1. Combine the ginger, shallots, vinegar, lemon juice, wine or soy sauce, salt, and oil in a blender. Puree until smooth. Season to taste with pepper. This dressing keeps, tightly sealed in a jar in the refrigerator, for up to 2 days.

Nutrient Analysis: Ginger Vinaigrette (1 tablespoon)

Calories	64
Protein	0.7 g
Carbohydrates	0.8 g
Fiber	0.0 g
Fat Total	7.0 g
Saturated	0.5 g
Mono	4.0 g
Poly Fat	2.0 g
Cholesterol	0.0 mg
Arginine	0.0 g

HERB-INFUSED OLIVE OIL

MAKES ½ CUP

6-inch sprig fresh rosemary
6 sprigs fresh oregano
4 sprigs fresh thyme
1 teaspoon whole black peppercorns (optional)
⅓ cup extra virgin olive oil

1. Bring a medium saucepan of water to a boil. Add the rosemary, oregano, thyme, and peppercorns, if you are using them. Boil 1 minute. Remove the herbs, using tongs. Shake the herbs, then pat dry in paper toweling.
2. Place the herbs and peppercorns in a small saucepan. Add the olive oil. Set over medium-low heat until bubbles just begin appearing around the edge of the oil. Remove from the heat.
3. Wash a small jar with a tight-fitting lid in very hot water. Dry it, using paper toweling. Using tongs, place the herbs and peppercorns in the jar. Add the oil. Cover and refrigerate at least 24 hours before using. The herbs can be left in the oil for up to 48 hours. After that, remove the herbs. This oil keeps up to a week, tightly covered, in the refrigerator. After that, it should be discarded to avoid the possible growth of harmful bacteria.

Nutrient Analysis: Herb-Infused Olive Oil (1 tablespoon)

Calories	37
Protein	0.0 g
Carbohydrates	0.0 g
Fiber	0.0 g
Fat Total	4.1 g
Saturated	0.6 g
Mono	3.2 g
Poly	0.4 g
Cholesterol	0.0 mg
Arginine	0.0 g

HONEY MUSTARD DRESSING
MAKES 3 TABLESPOONS

1 tablespoon honey mustard
1 tablespoon white wine vinegar
½ teaspoon salt, or to taste
1 tablespoon extra virgin olive oil

1. In a small bowl, whisk together the mustard, vinegar, and salt. Whisk in the oil. This dressing keeps 3 to 4 days, tightly covered in the refrigerator. Stir before using. Use as a sandwich spread as well as a dressing.

Calories	60
Protein	0.6 g
Carbohydrates	2.7 g
Fiber	0.3 g
Fat Total	5.6 g
Saturated	0.8 g
Mono	3.9 g
Poly Fat	0.9 g
Cholesterol	0.0 mg
Arginine	0.0 g

MANGO MINT SALSA

SERVES 4

½ large ripe mango
2 medium plum tomatoes, seeded and finely chopped
¼ poblano chili pepper or ¼ green bell pepper and 1 jalapeno
    pepper, finely chopped
¼ cup finely chopped red onion
½ cup chopped cilantro leaves, loosely packed
¼ cup chopped mint leaves, loosely packed
Juice of 1 lime
Salt and freshly ground pepper

1. Using a large spoon, scoop the flesh out of the mango. Chop it
   into small pieces; there should be about ⅔ cup. Place in a bowl.
2. Add the tomatoes, chili pepper, onion, cilantro, mint, and lime
   juice. Mix to combine. Season to taste with salt and pepper.

Calories	32
Protein	0.8 g
Carbohydrates	8.0 g
Fiber	1.2 g
Fat Total	0.2 g
Saturated	0.0 g
Mono	0.1 g
Poly	0.1 g
Cholesterol	0.0 mg
Arginine	0.0 g

VEGETABLES

BRAISED SWISS CHARD
SERVES 4

1 large bunch Swiss chard with white stems, washed and dried
1 tablespoon olive oil
2 large shallots, thinly sliced
2 tablespoons golden raisins
1½ cups defatted, low-sodium chicken stock or reduced-sodium
   canned broth
Salt and freshly ground black pepper to taste

1. Cut the stems off the chard at the base of the leaf and discard. Using a small knife, cut the stem out of the center of each leaf by running the knife down the sides of the stem, then detaching it at the top. Cut these stems crosswise into ½-inch slices and set aside.

2. Fold a leaf in half lengthwise, then roll it up from the bottom. Cut the roll crosswise into ½-inch strips. Repeat, slicing all the chard. There will be about 12 cups.

3. In a large skillet, heat the oil over medium-high heat. Add the shallots. Sauté until they are lightly browned. Remove with a slotted spoon and drain on paper toweling.

4. Add the sliced stems to the pan. Cook, stirring occasionally, for 2 minutes. Add half the remaining chard, stirring with a wooden spoon until it wilts, about 2 minutes. Add the rest of the chard and stir until wilted, 2 minutes. Add the raisins. Pour in the stock or broth. Simmer, uncovered, until the stems and chard are tender, 12 to 15 minutes, stirring occasionally. Serve hot or at room temperature. This side dish keeps, tightly covered in the refrigerator, for 2 to 3 days. Reheat in the microwave or simmer with a few tablespoons chicken broth, tightly covered over medium heat.

Nutrient Analysis: Braised Swiss Chard (1 serving)

Calories	102
Protein	4.3 g
Carbohydrates	12.4 g
Fiber	2.7 g
Fat Total	4.2 g
Saturated	0.6 g
Mono	2.7 g
Poly	0.4 g

Cholesterol	0.0 mg
Arginine	0.1 g

BROCCOLI WITH ROASTED GARLIC
SERVES 2

1 bunch broccoli
2 teaspoons extra virgin olive oil
3 to 5 roasted garlic cloves, peeled
Salt and freshly ground black pepper

1. Cut the broccoli into florets. Cut the tough outer peel away from the outside of the stems. Cut the tender inside of the stems crosswise into ¾-inch slices.
2. Cook the broccoli in a large pot of boiling water until it is just tender, 5 minutes. Drain well.
3. While the broccoli cooks, place oil in a medium nonstick skillet. Add the garlic. Set the pan over medium-high heat. Cook 2 minutes, mashing the garlic with a fork until it is pulpy and mixed with the oil.
4. Add the broccoli. Stir until the broccoli is coated with the oil and heated through. Season to taste with salt and pepper. Serve hot or lukewarm.

Nutrient Analysis: Broccoli with Roasted Garlic (1 serving)

Calories	99
Protein	7.1 g
Carbohydrates	13.6 g
Fiber	6.9 g
Fat Total	3.9 g
Saturated	0.6 g
Mono	2.4 g
Poly	0.7 g
Cholesterol	0.0 mg
Arginine	0.4 g

EGGPLANT, ZUCCHINI, AND TOMATO TIAN
SERVES 4

3 slices stale Italian peasant bread
½ teaspoon salt, divided
Freshly ground black pepper
1 small eggplant, cut diagonally into ½-inch slices
4 medium plum tomatoes, sliced
1 medium zucchini, cut diagonally into ½-inch slices
2 large garlic cloves, thinly sliced
2 tablespoons fresh thyme leaves
½ cup defatted, low-sodium chicken broth or vegetable broth
3 tablespoons extra virgin olive oil

1. Preheat the oven to 375°F. Rub a 9-inch × 13-inch lasagna pan with a bit of olive oil, or coat it with cooking spray, and set aside.
2. Break the bread up into 1-inch pieces. Whirl in the food processor to make ½ cup coarse bread crumbs. (If the bread is not stale, dry it out in a 300°F oven for about 10 minutes, taking care not to let it color.) In a small bowl, mix the bread crumbs with half the salt. Season liberally with freshly ground pepper.
3. Arrange the vegetables in a row, starting with an eggplant slice, a slice of tomato, and a zucchini slice, overlapping them to cover half the slice of vegetable underneath. Insert a sliver of the garlic between the eggplant and tomato. Continue, alternating slices of eggplant and zucchini, always placing a slice of tomato in between. Slip in slivers of garlic until it is all used. Sprinkle the thyme leaves over the layered vegetables. Pour on the broth. Sprinkle the seasoned bread crumbs over the vegetables. Drizzle with olive oil.
4. Bake uncovered, until the bread crumbs are crisp and browned and the vegetables are soft, about 30 minutes. Cool to room temperature and serve. This dish keeps at cool room temperature for up to 8 hours. It is best when made the day it is served, and not refrigerated.

Nutrient Analysis: Eggplant, Zucchini, and Tomato Tian (1 serving)

Calories	227
Protein	4.9 g
Carbohydrates	24.8 g
Fiber	5.3 g

Fat Total	13.2 g
Saturated	1.8 g
Mono	8.8 g
Poly	1.9 g
Cholesterol	0.0 mg
Arginine	0.1 g

GLAZED CARROTS

SERVES 2

2 teaspoons unsalted butter or canola oil
4 medium carrots, cut diagonally in ½-inch slices
⅔ cup freshly squeezed orange juice
Salt and freshly ground black pepper

1. Melt the butter in a medium, nonstick skillet over medium-high heat. Add the carrots, stirring to coat them with the butter. Cook 2 minutes.
2. Add the juice. Reduce the heat to medium and cook until the juice has evaporated and the carrots are still slightly crisp, about 10 minutes, stirring occasionally. Season to taste with salt and pepper and serve.

Nutrient Analysis: Glazed Carrots (1 serving)

Calories	91
Protein	1.1 g
Carbohydrates	13.4 g
Fiber	1.7 g
Fat Total	3.9 g
Saturated	2.7 g
Mono	0.0 g
Poly	0.1 g
Cholesterol	10.0 mg
Arginine	0.1 g

ROASTED ONIONS
SERVES 4 (MAKES 2 CUPS)

3 medium yellow onions
1 teaspoon finely chopped fresh rosemary
1 teaspoon finely chopped oregano leaves
2 teaspoons balsamic vinegar
1 tablespoon extra virgin olive oil
Salt and freshly ground black pepper

1. Preheat the oven to 500°F.
2. Line a baking dish just large enough to hold the onions with aluminum foil. Coat it with cooking spray. Remove only the loosest papery layers of the skin covering the onions. Place the onions, in their skin, in the pan. Add 1 cup water.
3. Bake the onions until they are very soft when pressed with a finger, 45 to 60 minutes. They will be very dark brown on the outside and blackened at the top. Set aside to cool.
4. When the onions are cool enough to handle, cut off their root end. Squeeze the soft flesh out onto a cutting board, leaving behind one or two of the outermost, tough layers just inside the skin. Coarsely chop the roasted onions and place in a small bowl. Mix the rosemary, oregano, vinegar, and oil into the onions. Season to taste with salt and pepper. Set aside, for 30 minutes, to allow flavors to develop. Or cover and refrigerate. These onions keep, tightly covered in the refrigerator, for up to 5 days.

Nutrient Analysis: Roasted Onions (½ cup)

Calories	78
Protein	1.5 g
Carbohydrates	10.9 g
Fiber	2.2 g
Fat Total	3.5 g
Saturated	0.5 g
Mono	2.7 g
Poly	0.3 g
Cholesterol	0.0 mg
Arginine	0.0 g

STIR-FRIED BABY BOK CHOY WITH GINGER
SERVES 4

16 to 24 baby bok choy (depending on size)
1 tablespoon peanut oil
2 teaspoons finely chopped fresh ginger
1 small garlic clove, halved
¼ cup defatted, low-sodium chicken or vegetable broth
3 or 4 drops roasted sesame oil
Freshly ground black pepper

1. Wash the bok choy carefully, swishing it in cold water to remove any grit and sand. Dry the bok choy well. Cut each cluster lengthwise in half.
2. Heat the peanut oil in a wok or large, heavy skillet over the highest possible heat. Add the ginger and garlic. Stir-fry until they are fragrant, 30 seconds. Add the bok choy. Stir-fry until the leaves wilt, 1 to 2 minutes. Add the broth. Stir-fry until the stems are tender-crisp, 2 to 3 minutes. Remove from the heat. Immediately add the sesame oil. Toss to coat the bok choy. Season with pepper to taste, and serve immediately.

Nutrient Analysis: Stir-Fried Baby Bok Choy with Ginger (1 serving)

Calories	59
Protein	2.9 g
Carbohydrates	4.2 g
Fiber	3.0 g
Fat Total	4.1 g
Saturated	0.7 g
Mono	1.7 g
Poly	1.4 g
Cholesterol	0.0 mg
Arginine	0.1 g

MAIN COURSES

CHICKEN WRAP WITH REFRIED BEANS
SERVES 1

⅓ cup warm Refried Beans (p. 134)
10-inch sprouted wheat or whole wheat tortilla
2 ounces sliced roasted chicken (3 or 4 thin slices)
1 tablespoon green salsa, lightly drained
¼ green bell pepper, cut in 4 strips
3 thin tomato slices (½ small tomato)
1 tablespoon cilantro leaves
1 tablespoon pepitas (roasted pumpkin seeds)

1. Spread the beans to cover the tortilla, leaving a ½-inch border around the edges. Arrange the chicken slices in a row across the center of the tortilla.
2. Dot the salsa over the chicken. Lay the pepper over the chicken. Line up the tomato slices over the pepper. Sprinkle on the cilantro and pepitas. Starting at the bottom, roll up the tortilla. Serve, accompanied by more of the beans and salsa, if desired.

Nutrient Analysis: Chicken Wrap with Refried Beans

Calories	415
Protein	30.7 g
Carbohydrates	54.6 g
Fiber	8.3 g
Fat Total	14.0 g
Saturated	2.7 g
Mono	5.1 g
Poly	5.0 g
Cholesterol	47.6 mg
Arginine	1.7 g

REFRIED BEANS

MAKES 1½ CUPS

2 tablespoons canola oil
¼ cup finely chopped red onion
1 large garlic clove, chopped
1 medium jalapeno pepper, seeded and finely chopped
1 teaspoon ground cumin
1 15-ounce can pinto beans, rinsed and drained
Salt and freshly ground black pepper to taste

1. In a medium skillet over medium-high heat, heat the oil. Sauté the onion, garlic, and pepper until the onion is soft, 4 minutes. Stir in the cumin until it smells fragrant, 30 seconds. Add the beans. Using the back of a wooden spoon, mash about half the beans. Cook, stirring until the mixture is creamy, 2 minutes. Season to taste with salt and pepper. Transfer to a bowl. These beans keep, tightly covered in the refrigerator, for 5 days.

Nutrient Analysis: Refried Beans (1½ cups)

Calories	532
Protein	20.5 g
Carbohydrates	67.4 g
Fiber	24.1 g
Fat Total	22.2 g
Saturated	1.5 g
Mono	12.0 g
Poly	7.8 g
Cholesterol	0.0 mg
Arginine	0.6 g

LINGUINI WITH ROASTED VEGETABLE SAUCE

SERVES 6

1 small eggplant (1 pound), unpeeled, cut in ½-inch cubes
1 medium onion, chopped
1 yellow bell pepper, chopped
3 tablespoons extra virgin olive oil
2 large garlic cloves, minced

1 28-ounce can fire-roasted or regular diced tomatoes
¼ teaspoon red pepper flakes
1 cup chopped arugula, loosely packed
Salt and freshly ground pepper
12 ounces whole wheat linguini

1. Preheat the oven to 450°F.
2. Place the eggplant, onion, and pepper on a nonstick cookie sheet with shallow sides. Drizzle on 2 tablespoons of the olive oil. Toss with your hands to coat the vegetables. Spread them in an even layer on the cookie sheet. Bake 10 minutes. Remove from the oven and stir well. Respread the vegetables. Bake an additional 10 minutes.
3. Heat the remaining oil in a large nonstick skillet over medium-high heat. Sauté the garlic 1 minute, taking care not to let it color. Add the roasted vegetables, the canned tomatoes with their liquid, and the pepper flakes. Bring to a boil, reduce the heat, and simmer until the sauce thickens but the vegetables still hold their shape, about 5 minutes. Stir in the arugula. Remove the pan from the heat. Season to taste with salt and pepper. This sauce tastes best when made ahead and reheated.
4. While the sauce cooks, or reheats, prepare the pasta according to package directions. Divide the cooked pasta among 6 plates. Top with the sauce and serve. Tightly covered, this sauce keeps up to 4 days in the refrigerator and freezes well. (To serve 1 or 2 people, use 2 ounces dried pasta per serving.)

Nutrient Analysis: Roasted Vegetable Sauce (1 serving)

Calories	124
Protein	2.4 g
Carbohydrates	14.2 g
Fiber	4.8 g
Fat Total	7.2 g
Saturated	1.0 g
Mono	5.4 g
Poly	0.7 g
Cholesterol	0.0 mg
Arginine	0.1 g

MEXICAN TOFU-STUFFED PITA

MAKES 2

1 whole wheat pita bread
2 large romaine lettuce leaves
1 2-ounce piece Mexican-flavored baked tofu, cut lengthwise
   into 6 strips (see note)
1 medium tomatillo, husked and thinly sliced
½ small green bell pepper, thinly sliced
¼ cup salsa, slightly drained
½ small Hass avocado, cut in 6 slices
10 to 12 cilantro sprigs

1. Preheat the oven to 350°F.
2. Warm the pita bread in the oven, 2 to 3 minutes.
3. Meanwhile, stack the lettuce leaves and roll them lengthwise. Shred the lettuce by cutting it crosswise into thin strips.
4. Cut the warm pita vertically in half. Open the pocket in each half. Line each one with a lettuce leaf. Place three of the tofu strips in each pita. Top each with half the tomatillo slices and green pepper. Add the salsa. Top with the avocado and cilantro sprigs. Serve immediately.

NOTE: Several companies make a Mexican-flavored baked tofu, including Azumaya, Nasoya, and White Wave.

Nutrient Analysis: Mexican Tofu-Stuffed Pita (1 serving)

Calories	226
Protein	9.6 g
Carbohydrates	26.6 g
Fiber	6.7 g
Fat Total	11.1 g
Saturated	1.6 g
Mono	5.5 g
Poly	2.8 g
Cholesterol	0.0 mg
Arginine	0.5 g

MOROCCAN RED SNAPPER

SERVES 4

1½ cups flatleaf parsley leaves, lightly packed
1½ cups cilantro leaves, lightly packed
4 roasted garlic cloves
2 teaspoons sweet paprika
1 teaspoon ground cumin
Juice of 1 medium lemon
Pinch of cayenne pepper
½ teaspoon salt
⅛ teaspoon freshly ground black pepper
½ cup extra virgin olive oil
1½ pounds red snapper fillet

1. Chop the parsley and cilantro finely; there will be ½ cup herbs. Place in a bowl. Mash the garlic to a paste and add to the herbs.
2. Add the paprika, cumin, lemon juice, cayenne, salt, and pepper. Whisk in the olive oil.
3. Preheat the oven to 400°F.
4. Place the fish in a shallow baking dish. Spoon ⅓ cup of the sauce over the fish. Let sit to marinate at room temperature for 20 minutes. Bake the fish until it flakes easily at the thickest point, 15 to 20 minutes, depending on the thickness of the fillet. Serve, passing the remaining sauce in a small bowl.

Nutrient Analysis: Moroccan Red Snapper (1 serving)

Calories	443
Protein	36.1 g
Carbohydrates	4.4 g
Fiber	1.3 g
Fat Total	30.6 g
Saturated	4.4 g
Mono	22.0 g
Poly	3.3 g
Cholesterol	62.9 mg
Arginine	2.1 g

RED PEPPERS STUFFED WITH
BARLEY AND BLACK BEANS

SERVES 4

2 cups defatted, low-sodium chicken or vegetable broth
½ cup pearl barley
4 medium red bell peppers
1 cup canned black beans, rinsed and drained
1 rib celery, finely chopped
1 small red onion, finely chopped
¾ cup defrosted frozen or canned corn kernels
1 tablespoon chopped mint
1 tablespoon chopped oregano
Salt and freshly ground black pepper
1 tablespoon Herb-Infused Olive Oil (p. 124) or plain extra
  virgin olive oil
1 tablespoon fresh lemon juice

1. Bring the broth to a boil in a deep saucepan. Add the barley. Cover and cook until the barley is tender, about 40 minutes. Uncover and set aside to cool slightly.
2. Preheat the oven to 400°F.
3. Cut off the top of each pepper, just below the curve at the top. Scoop out the seeds, taking care not to tear the peppers or make a hole in the bottom. Set aside.
4. In a medium bowl, using a fork, combine the barley, beans, celery, onion, corn, mint, and oregano. Season to taste with salt and pepper. Mix in the oil.
5. Pack the filling firmly into the peppers, mounding it slightly on top. Set the stuffed peppers in a shallow baking dish just large enough to hold them snuggled together, such as a 9-inch pie plate. Add ½ cup water to the pan. Set a square of foil over the peppers, arranging it to cover just their tops.
6. Bake until a sharp knife easily pierces the peppers and they still hold their shape, 35 to 40 minutes. Remove the foil and drizzle a quarter of the lemon juice over each pepper. Cool 20 minutes and serve. Or cool to room temperature, transfer to a plate, cover completely with foil, and refrigerate up to 24 hours before serving.

Nutrient Analysis: Red Peppers Stuffed with Barley and Black Beans (1 serving)

Calories	252
Protein	10.6 g
Carbohydrates	43.5 g
Fiber	9.7 g
Fat Total	5.1 g
Saturated	0.9 g
Mono	3.1 g
Poly	0.8 g
Cholesterol	0.0 mg
Arginine	0.5 g

SALADE NIÇOISE

SERVES 2

8 romaine lettuce leaves
1 6-ounce can water-packed albacore tuna, drained
1 large celery rib, thinly sliced
1 small green bell pepper, seeded and diced
½ cup cooked shelled edamame
1 hard-boiled egg white, chopped
2 large basil leaves, cut crosswise into thin strips
1 plum tomato, cut lengthwise into 4 wedges
2 tablespoons black Niçoise olives
4 anchovies, rinsed and dried (optional)
1 tablespoon red wine vinegar
½ teaspoon salt
1 garlic clove, minced
3 tablespoons extra virgin olive oil
Freshly ground black pepper

1. Tear the lettuce into bite-sized pieces. Arrange the lettuce on a large platter. Place the tuna on top of the lettuce, in the center of the plate.
2. Arrange the celery, pepper, and edamame over the lettuce around the tuna. Sprinkle the chopped egg white, then the basil, over the vegetables. Add the tomato wedges and olives. Drape the an-

chovies over the tomatoes, if using. At this point, the salad can be covered with plastic wrap and refrigerated for up to 2 hours.

3. For the dressing, whisk the vinegar and salt together in a small bowl. Add the garlic. Whisk in the oil until blended. Season to taste with pepper. Pour the dressing over the salad just before serving and toss.

Nutrient Analysis: Salade Niçoise (1 serving, not including optional anchovies)

Calories	456
Protein	32.4 g
Carbohydrates	15.1 g
Fiber	5.6 g
Fat Total	30.2 g
Saturated	4.4 g
Mono	19.2 g
Poly	5.3 g
Cholesterol	35.7 mg
Arginine	2.1 g

SMOKED SALMON ROULADES
SERVES 2, MAKES 4 PIECES

12-inch square lavash bread
2 tablespoons soy cream cheese or fat-free dairy cream cheese
1 tablespoon honey mustard
2 cups watercress sprigs, packed (about ½ bunch)
4 ounces thinly sliced smoked salmon
2 plum tomatoes
Freshly ground black pepper

1. Lay the square of lavash on a cutting board or counter. In a small bowl, mix together the cream cheese and mustard. Spread to cover the lavash.
2. Arrange the cress to cover the cream cheese spread. Lay the salmon slices to cover the cress. Using a serrated knife, cut the top off the tomatoes. Stand one on the cut side. Cut the tomato vertically into the thinnest possible slices. Slice the second tomato. Arrange the tomato slices over the salmon. Season with pepper.

Starting at the bottom, roll the filled bread up as tightly as possible.

3. Place the roulade on a sheet of plastic wrap. Tightly roll and seal it. Refrigerate 1 to 2 hours. Unwrap and cut the roulade crosswise into 4 pieces. Serve immediately.

Nutrient Analysis: Smoked Salmon Roulades (two roulades)

Calories	277
Protein	18.9 g
Carbohydrates	36.2 g
Fiber	2.8 g
Fat Total	6.3 g
Saturated	1.3 g
Mono	2.1 g
Poly	2.2 g
Cholesterol	14.2 mg
Arginine	0.8 g

SMOKED TURKEY WRAP WITH DRIED CRANBERRIES
SERVES 1

1 10-inch whole wheat or sprouted wheat tortilla
1½ tablespoons low-fat Thousand Island Dressing (see note)
2 red lettuce leaves
3 ounces smoked turkey (4 thin slices)
4 Fuji apple slices
2 thin slices navel orange
1 tablespoon pecans, chopped
2 teaspoons dried cranberries, coarsely chopped

1. Heat a heavy, medium skillet over medium-high heat. Place the tortilla in the dry skillet and heat for 1 minute. Turn and heat for 30 seconds. Place the tortilla on a cutting board or the counter.

2. Spread the dressing to cover the tortilla, leaving a 1-inch border around the edge. Arrange the lettuce to cover the entire tortilla. Arrange the turkey to cover the lettuce. Place the apple slices across the middle of the tortilla in a row. Lay the orange slices on top of the apple. Sprinkle the pecans and cranberries over the fruit. Lift up the tortilla from the bottom, rolling it as tightly as pos-

sible. Serve immediately or wrap tightly in plastic wrap and refrigerate up to 12 hours before serving.

NOTE: Thousand Island Dressing is 1 tablespoon low-fat or fat-free mayonnaise, 1 tablespoon chili sauce, and ½ teaspoon pickle relish.

Nutrient Analysis: Smoked Turkey Wrap with Dried Cranberries

Calories	314
Protein	19.0 g
Carbohydrates	39.2 g
Fiber	4.6 g
Fat Total	11.6 g
Saturated	1.9 g
Mono	3.8 g
Poly	2.4 g
Cholesterol	43.9 mg
Arginine	0.6 g

SOY-GLAZED SALMON

SERVES 4

1¼ cups pineapple juice
2¼ teaspoons soy sauce (can use reduced-sodium soy sauce)
1 teaspoon ginger juice (see note)
⅛ teaspoon freshly ground pepper
1 teaspoon peanut oil
4 6-ounce salmon steaks

1. Preheat the oven to 400°F.
2. In a stainless steel, glass, or enamel-lined saucepan, boil 1 cup of the pineapple juice until it is reduced to ½ cup, about 8 minutes. Remove the pot from the heat. Mix in 2 teaspoons of the soy sauce, the ginger juice, pepper, and the peanut oil.
3. Place the salmon steaks in one layer in a baking dish. Pour half the pineapple juice mixture over the fish. Bake the fish until it is done as you like it, about 12 minutes for ¾-inch-thick slices cooked until they are evenly pink all the way through. Remove from the oven and set aside. Discard the liquid in the pan.

4. Add the remaining pineapple juice to what remains in the pot. Boil until this liquid is syrupy, about 6 minutes. Add the remaining ¼ teaspoon of soy sauce.
5. Transfer a salmon steak to each of four dinner plates. Spoon a quarter of the hot soy glaze over each piece of fish and serve.

NOTE: For ginger juice, grate 1½ inches peeled fresh ginger on the finest possible grater. (A rasp or ginger grater from an Asian food store is ideal.) Place the grated ginger in a paper towel and squeeze it over a small bowl. Measure and use the juice.

Nutrient Analysis: Soy-Glazed Salmon (1 serving)

Calories	294
Protein	34.1 g
Carbohydrates	9.4 g
Fiber	0.0 g
Fat Total	11.9 g
Saturated	1.9 g
Mono	4.1 g
Poly	4.7 g
Cholesterol	93.6 mg
Arginine	2.0 g

TURKEY MEATLOAF

SERVES 8

1 pound ground turkey breast
1½ cups cooked long-grain brown rice
1 large leek, white part only, finely chopped
1 celery rib, finely chopped
1 large shallot, finely chopped
1 large garlic clove, finely chopped
1 large egg white
2 teaspoons curry powder
1 teaspoon ground paprika
1 teaspoon salt
¼ teaspoon freshly ground black pepper

Topping

¼ cup tomato sauce
2 teaspoons black bean sauce

1. Preheat the oven to 375°F. Coat a 1½-quart loaf pan with cooking spray.
2. Place the ground turkey in a large bowl. Add the rice, leek, celery, shallot, garlic, and egg white. Using a fork, mix until the ingredients are well blended. Mix in the curry powder, paprika, salt, and pepper. Pack the meatloaf firmly into the prepared pan. Cover it tightly with foil.
3. Bake the meatloaf for 40 minutes. In a small bowl, combine the tomato sauce and black bean sauce. Remove the meatloaf from the oven and uncover it. Spread the tomato mixture over the top of the meatloaf. Return it to the oven, uncovered. Bake until it feels firm when pressed in the center with your finger and a thermometer inserted into the center of the loaf registers 160°F.
4. Let the meatloaf sit at least 20 minutes before slicing. Or cool the meatloaf completely in the pan, turn it out, and refrigerate it, wrapped in foil. This meatloaf keeps up to 5 days in the refrigerator.

Nutrient Analysis: Turkey Meatloaf (1 serving)

Calories	162
Protein	17.9 g
Carbohydrates	14.0 g
Fiber	1.5 g
Fat Total	3.7 g
Saturated	0.1 g
Mono	0.4 g
Poly	0.4 g
Cholesterol	46.4 mg
Arginine	0.5 g

TURKEY AND SWISS SANDWICH
SERVES 1

4 teaspoons honey mustard
2 slices multigrain bread, toasted
1 large red lettuce leaf
2 ounces thinly sliced fresh turkey breast

1 ounce thinly sliced reduced-fat Swiss-style cheese
Freshly ground pepper
2 inches cucumber, peeled and thinly sliced
1 small tomato, thinly sliced

1. Spread half the mustard on each slice of toast. Fold the lettuce and place it on one slice of the bread. Add the turkey and Swiss cheese. Season with a few grinds of pepper. Add the cucumber and tomato. Top with the remaining slice of toast. Cut the sandwich vertically in half. Arrange the two halves on a plate and serve.

NOTE: If packing this sandwich, wrap it uncut. Cut it just before serving.

Nutrient Analysis: Turkey and Swiss Sandwich

Calories	373
Protein	29.7 g
Carbohydrates	44.3 g
Dietary Fiber	11.7 g
Fat Total	10.8 g
Saturated	2.6 g
Mono	3.0 g
Poly	3.1 g
Cholesterol	51.9 mg
Arginine	1.4 g

GRAINS AND LEGUMES

BROWN RICE AND RED LENTIL PILAF
SERVES 4

¼ cup sliced almonds
1 tablespoon extra virgin olive oil
1 small onion, finely chopped
¾ cup brown basmati rice, rinsed and drained
½ cup red lentils, rinsed and drained
¼ cup dried currants
¼ teaspoon ground turmeric
1 teaspoon salt
Freshly ground black pepper

1. Preheat the oven to 350°F. Spread the almonds in one layer on a baking sheet. Toast until they are lightly golden, about 10 minutes, stirring 3 or 4 times so the nuts color evenly. Set aside. This can be done up to a day ahead and the nuts stored in a tightly sealed container.
2. Heat the oil in a medium saucepan over medium-high heat. Sauté the onion until it is lightly browned, 8 minutes.
3. Add the rice, lentils, and 3 cups cold water. Add the currants, turmeric, and salt. Bring to a boil. Reduce the heat, cover tightly, and simmer until the rice is tender, 40 to 45 minutes. Let sit 5 minutes, off the heat. Season to taste with pepper. Serve hot or lukewarm, garnished with the almonds.

Nutrient Analysis: Brown Rice and Red Lentil Pilaf (1 serving)

Calories	357
Protein	11.7 g
Carbohydrates	59.9 g
Fiber	7.4 g
Fat Total	8.8 g
Saturated	1.2 g
Mono	3.2 g
Poly	0.8 g
Cholesterol	0.0 mg
Arginine	0.7 g

BROWN RICE PILAF WITH DILL
SERVES 4

1 tablespoon canola oil
1 small onion, finely chopped
1 cup brown basmati rice, rinsed and drained
2¼ cups defatted, low-sodium chicken or vegetable broth
⅓ cup chopped dill
2 tablespoons sliced almonds for garnish (optional)

1. Heat the oil in a deep saucepan over medium-high heat. Sauté the onion until it is browned, 6 to 7 minutes. Stir in the rice until it is coated with oil.

2. Add the broth. Bring the liquid to a boil. Cover the pot, reduce the heat, and cook until the rice is done, about 30 minutes. Let sit, off the heat, covered, for 10 minutes. Using a fork, stir in the chopped dill. Garnish with the almonds, if using, and serve.

Nutrient Analysis: Brown Rice Pilaf with Dill (1 serving, not including almonds)

Calories	165
Protein	6.4 g
Carbohydrates	15.6 g
Fiber	3.7 g
Fat Total	9.9 g
Saturated	1.9 g
Mono	2.8 g
Poly	4.6 g
Cholesterol	0.0 mg
Arginine	0.5 g

BULGUR PILAF

SERVES 4

¼ cup pine nuts
1 cup medium bulgur
2 cups chicken stock, defatted, low-sodium chicken broth, or
   vegetable broth
2 tablespoons extra virgin olive oil
1 small carrot, finely chopped
1 celery rib, finely chopped
1 small red onion, finely chopped
Grated zest and juice of ½ lemon
½ cup chopped flatleaf parsley leaves, lightly packed
Salt and freshly ground pepper

1. In a heavy, dry skillet, toast the pine nuts over medium-high heat, stirring constantly until they are lightly browned, about 4 minutes. Or the nuts can be roasted in a shallow pan, at 350°F, shaking the pan often until they are browned, 8 to 10 minutes. Set aside to cool. This can be done up to 2 days ahead and the nuts stored in a tightly closed container.

2. Place the bulgur in a medium bowl. Bring the stock or broth to a boil in a pan. Pour it over the bulgur. Let sit for 40 minutes.

3. Meanwhile, heat the oil in a medium skillet over medium-high heat. Sauté the carrot, celery, and onion just until the onion is translucent. The carrot and celery should still be firm. Add the cooked vegetables to the soaked bulgur. Mix in the lemon zest, juice, and parsley. Season to taste with salt and pepper. This dish can be served warm or at room temperature, like a salad.

Nutrient Analysis: Bulgur Pilaf (1 serving)

Calories	272
Protein	9.6 g
Carbohydrates	33.2 g
Fiber	8.3 g
Fat Total	12.6 g
Saturated	2.0 g
Mono	7.4 g
Poly	2.8 g
Cholesterol	0.0 mg
Arginine	0.6 g

TOMATO BRUSCHETTA

MAKES 2 PIECES

1 medium tomato, seeded and chopped
2 slices Whole Wheat Crostini (p. 153)
2 teaspoons Herb-Infused Olive Oil (p. 124)
Salt and freshly ground black pepper

1. Arrange the chopped tomato on the top of the crostini. Drizzle with the oil. Season to taste with the salt and pepper. Serve immediately.

NOTE: To make this bruschetta portable, toss the tomatoes and oil in a small container and cover tightly. Spoon the tomatoes onto the bread just before serving and season. (Salting the tomatoes ahead of time wilts them.)

Nutrient Analysis: Tomato Bruschetta (2 pieces)

Calories	252
Protein	6.6 g
Carbohydrates	32.4 g
Fiber	5.4 g
Fat Total	12.1 g
Saturated	1.9 g
Mono	8.2 g
Poly	1.6 g
Cholesterol	0.0 mg
Arginine	0.3 g

QUINOA WITH BROCCOLI, SWEET POTATO, AND SMOKED TOFU

SERVES 6

¾ cup quinoa
1 tablespoon extra virgin olive oil
1 medium onion, quartered and sliced crosswise
1 medium sweet potato (8 ounces), peeled, halved lengthwise,
    and cut in ½-inch slices
2 cups small broccoli florets or frozen chopped broccoli
½ cup chicken or vegetable broth
1 cup frozen or canned corn (drained)
8 ounces smoked tofu, cut in ½-inch cubes
Salt and freshly ground black pepper
¼ cup roasted pumpkin seeds

1. Rinse the quinoa very well in a strainer and drain. Place quinoa in a medium saucepan. Add 2¼ cups water and bring to a boil. Reduce the heat, cover tightly, and simmer until the quinoa is tender, about 15 minutes. Let sit, covered, for 10 minutes.

2. While the quinoa cooks, heat the oil in a medium, nonstick skillet over medium-high heat. Sauté the onion until it is lightly browned, 8 minutes, stirring often. Add the sweet potato and the broccoli, if fresh. Pour in the chicken broth. Cover and cook until the potatoes are almost tender, about 5 minutes. If using frozen broccoli, add it at this point, along with the corn and tofu. Cover and cook until the potatoes are almost soft, but still hold their

shape, about 5 minutes. Stir in the cooked quinoa. Season to taste with salt and pepper. Serve hot, in shallow, wide soup bowls, garnished with the pumpkin seeds.

Nutrient Analysis: Quinoa with Broccoli, Sweet Potato, and Smoked Tofu (1 serving)

Calories	234
Protein	13.9 g
Carbohydrates	32.0 g
Fiber	5.0 g
Fat Total	6.5 g
Saturated	0.9 g
Mono	2.6 g
Poly	2.2 g
Cholesterol	0.0 g
Arginine	0.5 g

RED LENTILS WITH BEETS AND TOFU "FETA"
SERVES 4

3 small beets, scrubbed
1 cup Pickled Pressed Tofu (p. 151)
1 cup red lentils, rinsed and drained
½ medium cucumber, peeled, seeded, and diced
¼ cup snipped chives
2 tablespoons red wine vinegar
1 teaspoon ground cumin
½ teaspoon dried oregano
3 tablespoons extra virgin olive oil
Salt and freshly ground black pepper

1. Preheat the oven to 375°F.
2. Wrap the beets in aluminum foil. Set on the rack in the center of the oven. Bake until a knife easily pierces the center of the beets, about 40 minutes. Set aside to cool. Slip off the skin, using your fingers. Dice the beets and place in a medium bowl. Add the crumbled Pickled Pressed Tofu. Set aside.
3. Place the red lentils in a medium saucepan. Add cold water to a level that is 2 inches above the lentils. Cook over high heat until

the water boils. Reduce the heat and simmer until the lentils are still slightly firm in the center, 8 minutes. Drain the lentils in a strainer and place them in a medium bowl. Add the cucumber and 3 tablespoons of the chives to the hot lentils.

4. In a small bowl, whisk together the vinegar, cumin, oregano, and oil. Season to taste with salt and pepper. Pour half the vinaigrette over the lentils and half over the beets and tofu. Toss each to blend.

5. To serve, divide the lentils among four plates, making a bed of them on each. Heap a quarter of the beet mixture in the center. Garnish each plate with a quarter of the remaining chives.

Nutrient Analysis: Red Lentils with Beets and Tofu "Feta" (1 serving)

Calories	333
Protein	18.3 g
Carbohydrates	35.7 g
Fiber	10.1 g
Fat Total	14.1 g
Saturated	2.0 g
Mono	8.8 g
Poly	2.9 g
Cholesterol	0.0 mg
Arginine	1.3 g

PICKLED PRESSED TOFU
MAKES 1 1/2 CUPS

8 ounces (½ package) firm regular tofu, in one slab (see note)
½ teaspoon salt
2 tablespoons distilled white vinegar

1. Cover a cutting board with a sheet of plastic wrap. Place the tofu on the plastic wrap. Set another sheet of plastic wrap on top of the tofu. Place a second cutting board on top of the tofu. Arrange weights, such as a couple of large cans of tomatoes or a cast-iron skillet, on top of the cutting board, making sure the weight is evenly distributed. Let the weighted tofu sit for 45 minutes.

2. Remove the weights. Blot the tofu with paper toweling to dry it.

This pressed tofu will keep, submersed in cold water, for 3 to 4 days. Change the water daily.

3. To pickle the tofu, crumble it into a small bowl until it resembles large-curd cottage cheese, pulling it apart with your fingers. Add the salt and vinegar. Stir gently with a fork. Cover the bowl with plastic wrap and refrigerate for 30 minutes. The tofu can be kept up to 24 hours, covered in the refrigerator. It becomes more sharp and salty the longer it sits. Use this tofu crumbled over salads.

NOTE: Use tofu sold in a plastic tub or pouch, not the kind in a box. (See p. 70 for more information on types of tofu.)

Nutrient Analysis: Pickled Pressed Tofu (1 cup, as used in Red Lentils with Beets and Tofu "Feta")

Calories	219
Protein	23.9 g
Carbohydrates	6.5 g
Fiber	3.5 g
Fat Total	13.2 g
Saturated	1.9 g
Mono	2.9 g
Poly	7.4 g
Cholesterol	0.0 mg
Arginine	1.6 g

SOY TRAIL MIX
SERVES 8

½ cup whole salted soynuts
½ cup roasted sunflower seeds
¼ cup sliced almonds
¼ cup miniature chocolate chips
¼ cup raisins
1 slice unsulfured dried pineapple, cut in ¼-inch pieces

1. Combine the soybeans, sunflower seeds, almonds, chocolate chips, raisins, and chopped pineapple in a bowl. Transfer to an airtight container. Store in a cool, dry place for up to 2 weeks.

Nutrient Analysis: Soy Trail Mix (¼ cup)

Calories	165
Protein	6.4 g
Carbohydrates	15.6 g
Fiber	3.7 g
Fat Total	9.9 g
Saturated	1.9 g
Mono	2.8 g
Poly	4.6 g
Cholesterol	0.0 mg
Arginine	0.5 g

WHOLE WHEAT CROSTINI
MAKES 16

1 12-inch loaf Italian whole wheat bread (see note)
2 garlic cloves, halved (optional)
½ teaspoon extra virgin olive oil or Herb-Infused Olive Oil
(optional)

1. Place a rack in the center of the oven. Preheat the oven to 350°F.
2. Cut the bread diagonally into ½-inch slices.
3. Arrange the bread directly on the rack in the oven. Toast 5 minutes, until the bread turns light, golden brown around the edges. Remove from the oven with tongs and cool on a rack; the crostini become hard and crisp as they cool. These crostini keep, sealed in an airtight container, for one week.
4. If desired, just before serving, rub each crostini with one of the garlic halves, and/or drizzle with ½ teaspoon extra virgin olive oil or Herb-Infused Olive Oil (p. 124).

NOTE: A round, peasant-style or sourdough whole wheat loaf can also be used. Do not use a baguette or multigrain bread, as they do not toast to the right crispness.

Nutrient Analysis: Whole Wheat Crostini (2 crostini, not including the oil)

Calories	141
Protein	5.6 g
Carbohydrates	26.4 g
Dietary Fiber	3.9 g
Fat Total	2.4 g
Saturated	0.5 g
Mono	1.0 g
Poly	0.6 g
Cholesterol	0.0 mg
Arginine	0.3 g

WHOLE WHEAT PITA CRISPS

SERVES 1

1 whole wheat pita bread
1 garlic clove, halved
2 teaspoons extra virgin olive oil or Herb-Infused Olive Oil
    (p. 124)
¼ teaspoon salt (optional)

1. Place a rack in the center of the oven. Preheat the oven to 350°F.
2. Separate the pita into two rounds by working a small, sharp knife around the edge, then pulling the two halves apart using your fingers.
3. Rub each half with one of the garlic halves. Brush each half with 1 teaspoon of the oil. Stack the two halves. Cut the pita crosswise twice, quartering it, making 8 pieces in all. If desired, sprinkle a few grains of the salt on each piece.
4. Arrange the pita pieces in one layer on a baking sheet. Bake 4 to 5 minutes, until slightly darkened in color. Cool on the baking sheet; the Pita Crisps crisp as they cool.

NOTE: As an option, sprinkle 1½ tablespoons shredded Parmigiano-Reggiano cheese over the 8 pieces of pita before baking.

Nutrient Analysis: Whole Wheat Pita Crisps (1 whole pita crisp)

Calories	259
Protein	6.5 g
Carbohydrates	36.2 g
Fiber	4.8 g
Fat Total	11.0 g
Saturated	1.6 g
Mono	7.4 g
Poly	1.5 g
Cholesterol	0.0 mg
Arginine	0.3 g

DESSERTS

CHERRY BERRY COMPOTE
SERVES 4

1 12-ounce bag frozen unsweetened black cherries
1½ cups frozen unsweetened blueberries
1½ cups frozen unsweetened raspberries
2 tablespoons sugar
2 whole star anise, ¼ teaspoon Chinese five-spice powder, or a
*   4-inch cinnamon stick*

1. Place the cherries in a medium bowl and let sit, at room temperature, until defrosted, about 1 hour.
2. Place the blueberries, raspberries, sugar, and pieces of anise in a deep saucepan over medium-low heat. Stir to coat the fruit with the sugar. Cook gently until the sugar melts and some liquid appears, about 10 minutes. Raise the heat to medium and simmer, uncovered, until the blueberries are soft but still hold their shape and the raspberries are falling apart, 8 to 10 minutes. Pour the hot fruit over the cherries. Set aside to cool.
3. When the compote is cool, remove the anise. Serve at room temperature or chilled, ladled over ice cream or in a bowl with a dollop of vanilla yogurt. This compote keeps, tightly covered in the refrigerator, for 5 days.

Nutrient Analysis: Cherry Berry Compote (1 serving, not including ice cream or yogurt)

Calories	66
Protein	0.8 g
Carbohydrates	16.5 g
Fiber	3.3 g
Fat Total	0.4 g
Saturated	0.0 g
Mono	0.0 g
Poly	0.1 g
Cholesterol	0.0 mg
Arginine	0.0 g

CHOCOLATE RASPBERRY SURPRISE
SERVES 4

*6 ounces best-quality dark chocolate, finely chopped (not
   chocolate chips)*
1 cup (8 ounces) pureed silken tofu, at room temperature
1 teaspoon vanilla
½ cup fresh raspberries
4 mint sprigs, for garnish

1. For the chocolate mousse, melt the chocolate in a bowl over barely simmering water or in the microwave. Let the chocolate cool to lukewarm. Using a rubber spatula, stir the tofu and vanilla into the chocolate.

2. Spoon half the mousse into 4 dessert dishes or large wineglasses, dividing it evenly among them. Carefully spoon a quarter of the raspberries into the center of the mousse. Spoon in the remaining mousse, arranging it to cover the berries. Refrigerate until chilled, 2 hours. Let sit at room temperature 15 minutes before serving. The mousse keeps in the refrigerator, covered, for at least 3 days. It is best to assemble this dessert the day it will be served. Garnish with the mint before serving.

Nutrient Analysis: Chocolate Raspberry Surprise (1 serving)

Calories	252
Protein	4.4 g
Carbohydrates	28.5 g
Fiber	3.2 g
Fat Total	14.1 g
Saturated	8.6 g
Mono	4.9 g
Poly	0.9 g
Cholesterol	0.4 mg
Arginine	0.7 g

DOUBLE CHOCOLATE CAKE
SERVES 9

1¼ cups all-purpose flour
¼ cup toasted soy flour (see p. 100 for how to toast soy flour)
6 tablespoons Dutch-processed cocoa
¾ teaspoon baking soda
1 cup sugar
Pinch of salt
1 cup cold water
¼ cup canola oil
1 tablespoon white vinegar
2 teaspoons vanilla extract

Chocolate Ganache (Frosting)

3 ounces dark chocolate, chopped
¼ cup silken tofu, pureed (see p. 70 for information on types of
tofu)
½ teaspoon vanilla

1. Set a rack in the center of the oven. Preheat the oven to 350°F. Coat an 8-inch × 8-inch baking pan with cooking spray and flour it.
2. Sift the flour, soy flour, cocoa, and baking soda into a medium bowl. Whisk in the sugar and salt.
3. Combine the water, oil, vinegar, and vanilla. Pour them into the dry ingredients. Mix until the batter is smooth and silky, working

out most of the lumps with the back of a wooden spoon. Pour the batter into the prepared pan.

4. Bake 30 minutes, until the cake pulls away from the sides of the pan and a bamboo skewer inserted into the center comes out clean. Let the cake cool in the pan for 10 minutes. Turn it out onto a baking rack and cool completely.

5. For the ganache frosting, melt the chocolate in a small bowl in the microwave or over hot water in a double boiler. Let it cool to luke-warm. Puree the tofu in a miniature food processor or a blender. Add the tofu to the chocolate. Stir in the vanilla.

6. Spread the chocolate ganache evenly over the top of the cake. Serve while the frosting is creamy or refrigerate to set the frosting. Cut the cake into 9 squares and serve. This cake keeps, covered with foil, in the refrigerator for up to 3 days.

Nutrient Analysis: Double Chocolate Cake (1 serving)

Calories	266
Protein	4.4 g
Carbohydrates	41.6 g
Fiber	2.7 g
Fat Total	10.3 g
Saturated	2.7 g
Mono	3.9 g
Poly	2.1 g
Cholesterol	0.0 mg
Arginine	0.1 g

RED GRAPE MACÉDOINE

SERVES 4

½ cup sugar
1 3-inch cinnamon stick
1 whole star anise
3 strips lemon zest, ½ inch × 2 inches
3 strips lime zest, ½ inch × 2 inches
3 strips orange zest, 1 inch × 2 inches
1½ cups seedless red grapes, halved
1 cup fresh blueberries

½ cup fresh raspberries
½ cup fresh blackberries, red currants, or gooseberries (see note)
½ cup light, dry red wine, such as Beaujolais

1. Place the sugar in a heavy, medium saucepan. Add ½ cup cold water. Add the cinnamon, star anise, and lemon, lime, and orange zests. Set the pan over medium-high heat. When the sugar has dissolved and the syrup comes come to a boil, cover the pot and remove it from the heat. Let the syrup sit, covered, for 30 minutes. Remove the spices and zest, reserving the zest. Let the syrup cool to room temperature.
2. Place the grapes, blueberries, raspberries, and blackberries, currants, or gooseberries in a clear glass serving bowl. Pour in the syrup. Mix in the red wine. Cut the reserved citrus zest crosswise into very thin strips. Sprinkle the zest over the fruit salad. Cover with plastic wrap and refrigerate 1 hour to let the flavors blend. Serve in bowls, spooning a generous amount of the liquid over the fruit. Red Grape Macédoine keeps up to 24 hours, tightly covered, in the refrigerator.

NOTE: If blackberries or other suggested fruit are not available, increase amount of raspberries to 1 cup. Do not use frozen fruit.

Nutrient Analysis: Red Grape Macédoine (1 serving)

Calories	200
Protein	1.0 g
Carbohydrates	46.1 g
Fiber	4.1 g
Fat Total	0.6 g
Saturated	0.1 g
Mono	0.0 g
Poly	0.2 g
Cholesterol	0.0 mg
Arginine	0.1 g

SOY'MORES

SERVES 4

1 ounce good-quality dark chocolate, coarsely chopped
2 whole wheat honey-sweetened graham crackers (4 squares)
4 tablespoons soynut butter

1. Place the chocolate in a small, microwavable bowl. Melt the chocolate, uncovered, in the microwave oven, about 30 seconds. Stir it and set aside.
2. Break each cracker into 2 squares. Spread each cracker with 1 tablespoon of the soynut butter, making a thick layer.
3. Spread a quarter of the chocolate over each cracker, bringing it down to the edge of the cracker to cover the soynut butter completely. Place the Soy'mores on a plate or baking sheet.
4. To set the chocolate, refrigerate the Soy'mores for about 10 minutes. Serve or cover with plastic wrap and refrigerate. Soy'mores keep for 3 days in the refrigerator. Let them sit at room temperature for at least 15 minutes before serving.

Nutrient Analysis: Soy'mores (1 serving)

Calories	149
Protein	4.4 g
Carbohydrates	14.4 g
Fiber	2.3 g
Fat Total	8.3 g
Saturated	2.4 g
Mono	1.4 g
Poly	4.0 g
Cholesterol	0.3 mg
Arginine	0.2 g

SUMMER FRUIT SALAD

SERVES 4

½ ripe papaya
1 kiwi fruit, yellow or green, peeled, halved, and sliced
1 peach or nectarine, thinly sliced
½ pint (1 cup) fresh blueberries
1 cup fresh raspberries
Juice of ½ lime

1. Leave the fruit out until it is room temperature, about 30 minutes.
2. Scoop the seeds out of the papaya. Cut it lengthwise into 3 pieces. Slice the flesh away from the skin. Cut the papaya crosswise into 1-inch pieces. Place in a medium bowl.
3. Add the kiwi, peach, blueberries, raspberries, and lime juice to the bowl. Toss with a fork to avoid bruising the fruit. Serve at room temperature.

Nutrient Analysis: Summer Fruit Salad (1 serving)

Calories	70
Protein	1.4 g
Carbohydrates	20.3 g
Fiber	6.0 g
Fat Total	0.4 g
Saturated	0.1 g
Mono	0.1 g
Poly	0.0 g
Cholesterol	0.0 mg
Arginine	0.0 g

A GLASS OF WINE

A 4- to 5-ounce glass of wine is about 100 to 120 calories. Drink in moderation and try to balance your caloric intake accordingly. You may want to skip dessert or forgo the flatbread crackers when you have wine.

Chapter 6

Exercise and the Endothelium

BEING PHYSICALLY active on a regular basis is simply one of the best things you can do for your heart and vessels. No matter how old you are, you can always improve your health by being active.

Despite our knowledge of the benefits of exercise and health, most Americans don't incorporate physical activity into their lives. Granted, there are fewer opportunities to be active now than there were in past eras. Our jobs are often sedentary. There is television watching, driving around in cars, and relying on machines to do chores around the house. Thus, in this day and age, physical activity takes an effort. If more people understood how much this effort would help their health, perhaps more would join in.

About 88 million Americans are inactive, according to the American Council on Exercise. In 1997, only 22 percent of Americans were active enough to benefit from their physical activity. And the Centers for Disease Control and Prevention is so concerned about the 34 percent of the adult population over 50 who are sedentary that in 2001 they released *National Blueprint: Increasing Physical Activity Among Adults Aged 50 and Older,* a report that strongly recommends that this segment of the population boost its physical activity.

The problem is even extending to our children, who are more overweight and less active than any other generation of children. In 1999, researchers found that 60 percent of 5- to 10-year-old children had at least one risk for heart disease, including high blood lipids, elevated blood pressure, or elevated insulin levels. This striking increase in the number of children with risk factors is due in large part to less physical activity and increased body weight.

Heart Health Benefits of Aerobic Exercise

PHYSICAL ACTIVITY improves overall health, and cardiovascular health in particular. It helps you steer free of cardiovascular disease or helps you manage the disease if you have it. By contrast, couch potatoes are at increased risk for heart attack and stroke.

Aerobic exercise is the best way to enhance cardiovascular fitness. This form of exercise specifically benefits the heart and blood vessels and makes the whole cardiovascular system work more efficiently. Brisk walking, jogging, jumping rope, cross-country skiing, dancing, swimming, and biking are all examples of this type of exercise; they all involve exertion that requires vigorous and sustained activity of the large muscle groups.

(The other two types of exercise are strength training to improve muscle strength and stretching to improve flexibility of the joints. Strength training, particularly with heavy weights and few repetitions, does not improve cardiovascular fitness and could even be detrimental. [See Should You Lift Weights?, p. 170.] By contrast, stretching is an important part of an aerobic exercise program. After your workout, when your muscles are well warmed up, it's a good idea to stretch them as part of your cool-down. (See more about cooling down on p. 173.)

Aerobic exercise has a number of beneficial metabolic effects that prevent heart disease. It reduces LDL (bad) cholesterol and increases HDL (good) cholesterol. Regular exercise also reduces your blood sugar to healthy levels and lowers blood pressure and heart rate. Because of these beneficial effects, exercise can slow or even reverse hardening of the arteries.

Aerobic exercise burns calories—and is thus, along with modifying your food intake, one of the most useful ways of decreasing total body fat. This is important for a number of reasons. Carrying around extra weight contributes to several types of disease, including heart disease, high blood pressure, stroke, and diabetes. By maintaining a healthy weight, you are much more likely to remain disease free.

As for other aspects of health, aerobic exercise provides a number of other benefits: it reduces stress, depression, and anxiety; improves sleep; improves immune function; enhances mood and self-image; boosts stamina and energy; and increases life span.

A More Efficient Heart

THE HEART is a muscle and, like all the other muscles in your body, can be strengthened and made stronger with exercise. When you exercise regularly, the work of the heart becomes more efficient. The result is a heart that beats less often, and works less hard, to do the job of delivering oxygen to working muscles.

People who are active and whose hearts work efficiently have low heart rates when they are at rest. The normal range of resting heart rate for an adult is between 60 and 90 beats per minute. As I am typing this, my resting heart rate is 58.

To figure out your resting heart rate while you read this, take your pulse. The best way to do this is at the wrist. Turn the left hand palm up (if you are left-handed, take the pulse at the right wrist). Place your first two fingers on your wrist right below the base of the thumb. Move these fingers around on the wrist until you feel the pulse. Count for 15 seconds and then multiply by four to find out how many times your heart beats in a minute.

Obviously, it is healthier to have a heart rate in the lower range of normal (a good resting heart rate is between 60 and 70). Some people in very good physical shape have heart rates that are even lower; for example, endurance athletes can have resting heart rates as low as 36.

(Note that if you are above the age of 40, have a heart rate less than 60, *and are not physically fit,* this may be abnormal. Your doctor can quickly determine if there is a problem with an EKG.)

However, if your resting heart rate is in the 90 to 100 range, you have an increased risk of heart attack and stroke. The Chicago Heart Association Detection Project in Industry studied over 30,000 employees of companies and organizations in the Chicago area for over 20 years. One of the things gleaned from this study was that a resting heart rate that was 12 beats per minute more than normal (a heart rate that was about 100 beats per minute) increased risk of heart attack, stroke, and death by about 10 percent.

That daily exercise reduces your chance of heart attack has been well documented in a number of studies. For example, in the Honolulu Heart Program, begun in 1965 by the National Heart, Lung, and Blood Institute, 8,000 Hawaiian men of Japanese ancestry were carefully monitored by researchers for 30 years. The researchers found that retired men who walked two miles daily had half the risk of having serious heart disease than those who were sedentary.

Regular exercise also reduces your chance of a stroke. In the 1999 Reykjavik Study, Iceland researchers studied 4,500 middle-aged men for 10 years. The men who continued to exercise regularly after the age of 40 had about 30 percent fewer strokes during that period of time than those who didn't exercise.

Aerobic Exercise and the Endothelium

AEROBIC EXERCISE enhances your heart and vessel health by providing direct benefit to the endothelium. In fact, one of the best things you can do to have or restore a healthy endothelium is to be active.

When you exercise, the flow of blood through your vessels increases. The endothelium can sense this increase in flow and, in response, makes NO. Your vessels react to NO by opening up to accommodate the increased flow of blood.

When you exercise, your vessels make more of the enzyme NO synthase. The body produces NO with the help of the enzyme NO synthase. By exercising, you boost your vessels' production of NO synthase, the factory in the body where NO is made.

When you exercise, you improve the Teflon-like quality of the endothelium. When endothelial cells are exposed to long-term increases in flow, they become less sticky and more like Teflon. White blood cells and platelets are less likely to cling to the vessel, and plaque is less likely to build up in the arteries. This might explain why people who exercise regularly are less likely to have a heart attack. Researchers at Stanford and elsewhere have used angiography to study the long-term effects of exercise on the coronary arteries. They have observed that heart patients who exercise regularly have fewer blockages in their heart arteries. Furthermore, people who exercise regularly have coronary arteries that relax much more than the arteries of couch potatoes.

When you exercise, you increase the diameter of your blood vessels. The great cardiac pathologist Paul Wood first noted this about 60 years ago when he did an autopsy on an old marathon runner who had died of cancer. Dr. Wood observed that the coronary arteries of the "marathon man" were two to three times the size of a normal man. Since then, a number of investigators have shown that exercise causes vessels to remodel in a positive way. Vessels actually change their structure in response to long-term increases in blood flow—their diameter increases. More recently, researchers at Stanford have observed that in middle-aged ultra-distance marathon runners, the heart arteries have twice the capacity to open up than those of sedentary people of the same age and gender.

When you exercise, you counter the normal process of aging and its impact on blood vessels. Researchers have noted that people who participate in aerobic exercise have improved endothelial health, regardless of their age. For example, one result of aging is a diminished supply of NO released from the endothelium. But exercise seems to change that process. A study from the University of Pisa found that blood vessels of very active older people (their average age was 63) functioned just as well as blood vessels of athletes half their age. Even for people who have been sedentary, daily light to moderate exercise will improve endothelial health and reduce risk of cardiovascular disease.

These beneficial effects of exercise on the endothelium can occur in people with heart disease. Even in people with disease of the heart arteries, regular exercise improves blood flow through the heart muscle and improves delivery of oxygen and nutrients. Drs. Rainer Hambrecht and Anamaria Wolf at the University of Leipzig Heart Center in Germany have shown that a four-week exercise program improved endothelial function in patients with coronary artery disease. Even in diseased arteries, exercise enhanced the production of NO, which enabled the vessels to accommodate an increased flow of blood. This demonstrates that the endothelium can rapidly respond to exercise.

When I was at the Mayo Clinic, I saw a lawyer who was having a lot of trouble walking because of poor circulation in his legs. During a treadmill test, it was clear that he had no problem with his heart but had pretty severe hardening of the arteries affecting the vessels to his legs. He could walk only half a block before he developed pain. Overweight and sedentary, he had no discomfort most of the time because he avoided walking. I put him on an exercise program and asked him to start by taking a 20-minute walk every day. I told him to walk until his legs got tired, rest, and then continue walking until he had completed 20 minutes. After two weeks, I asked him to increase the duration of his walk by 5 minutes. I kept asking him to increase his walk by 5 minutes every two weeks until he was taking a 45-minute walk daily. When he came back to see me three months later, he was dramatically improved and was able to walk two miles without stopping.

What happened to this lawyer that had allowed him to improve so much? Well, for one thing, the increase in exercise caused him to burn more calories, and he lost some weight. As you might expect, it is easier to walk farther when carrying less weight. In addition, some interesting things happen to your circulation when you walk regularly. Your vascular production of nitric oxide improves, and the vessels are able to relax better. You develop biological bypasses around blocked vessels. These "collateral" vessels are small, and although they cannot handle as much blood flow as a normal vessel, exercise makes them larger over time. The enlarged collateral vessels can supply more blood flow to the leg (or heart if the blockage is in the heart arteries). Furthermore, with regular exercise, the muscle becomes much better at using the available blood flow. Drs. Bill Hiatt and Judith Regensteiner at the University of Colorado have found that regular exercise enhances the cellular machinery necessary to burn fat and sugar and turn nutrients into energy. Therefore, regular exercise can improve blood flow to the skeletal and heart muscles and can improve the functioning of these muscles.

How Much Exercise Do You Need— the Current Recommendations

THE GOOD news about exercise is that you don't have to be a marathon runner to reap the benefits. A moderate amount of exercise daily will prolong your life. But just how much do you need? There has been much speculation and research on this question, as well as a host of varying guidelines.

It was noted in the *Harvard Women's Health Watch* that perhaps the lack of activity in America is due to confusion and a "lack of specifics."[1] In the 1970s and 1980s, the message about exercise was "no pain, no gain." It was believed that unless you exercised vigorously, you simply did not reap the benefits. But by the mid-1990s, experts realized that the "vigorous" message was leaving much of the public behind.

In 1996, the U.S. Department of Health and Human Services issued "Physical Activity and Health: A Report of the Surgeon General," the first report of its kind to recommend exercise to adults. The report urged that adults accumulate 30 minutes or more of moderate-intensity physical activity on most, if not all, days of the week. This recommendation differed from others that had come before it since it emphasized moderate exercise (30 minutes most days of the week) as opposed to vigorous.

In one of the most recent studies, researchers at Harvard Medical School have found that women can reduce their risk of cardiovascular disease by walking for one hour a week. The researchers evaluated data from the Women's Health Study, a randomized, double-blind, placebo-controlled trial of low-dose aspirin and vitamin E for prevention of cardiovascular disease. The 40,000 women, ages 45 and over, answered questions about their daily physical activity. Keeping in mind risk factors for cardiovascular disease, such as smoking, weight, diet, and family history, the researchers determined that as little as one hour of casual weekly walking lowered risk of coronary heart disease. Other research shows that the more exercise you do, the better off you are. But this new contribution from Harvard is a boon to sedentary women—that just one hour of walking per week reduces heart disease.

So, how much should you exercise? The answer depends on how fit you are right now. Recognizing this, the current American Heart Association recommendations for physical activity are divided into two groups.

For individuals who already exercise, the recommendation is:
Perform vigorous aerobic exercise for at least 30 minutes, three to four days a week at 50 to 75 percent of your maximum heart rate. (See the Target Heart Rate table, p. 169.)

Moderate activity lasting for 30 minutes on most days also provides some benefit.

For individuals who are sedentary or unable to exercise vigorously, the recommendation is:
Do as much moderate or low-intensity aerobic exercise as you can. Even a small amount can help lower the risk of cardiovascular disease. I recommend walking for at least 30 minutes daily. Participate in recreational activities. Even low-intensity activities such as gardening and housework count. Do some form of physical activity

every day and I guarantee that your heart and vessels will be healthier. (For more information on walking, see p. 172.)

If you are starting an exercise program for the first time or after having been inactive for a long time, see my recommendations on p. 171 for what beginners should do before they start an exercise program.

TARGET HEART RATE

Use the following equation to calculate the maximum heart rate for your age group:

220 - age = maximum heart rate (MAX HR)

This number is your maximum heart rate (MAX HR), which represents your heart rate if you exercised to your utmost ability. Your maximum heart rate is the first number you need to determine a safe, and challenging, Target Heart Rate for your fitness level. The Target Heart Rate is the heart rate that you wish to reach during exercise and maintain for at least 20 minutes.

- If you are already active, multiply your MAX HR by 75 percent to obtain your Target Heart Rate. The body's heart, lungs, and circulation system all benefit when you exercise at this heart rate.

- If you have been sedentary but otherwise feel fine and are at low risk for heart disease, multiply your MAX HR by 60 percent to obtain your Target Heart Rate. After you have been exercising regularly at this Target Heart Rate for a few weeks, you can increase your Target Heart Rate to about 75 percent of your MAX HR.

- The above formula is not as useful over age 65. Over age 65, I think it is reasonable to aim for a target HR of 100 if you have been sedentary, and increase up to 115 as your body becomes more conditioned to exercise. Some very fit individuals in the older age groups can exercise at a target HR above this level.

- If you are at high risk for heart disease, and particularly if you have symptoms, see your doctor before beginning an exercise program. You may need to have an EKG-monitored treadmill test to determine a safe level of exercise.

How to use your Target Heart Rate when you exercise:
When you exercise (for example, go for a 30-minute walk), start out slowly and increase your pace over a 10-minute period until you are exercising at a level that you feel has increased your pulse and breathing rate. Check your pulse at this point. (See p. 164 for information on how to do this.) Try to achieve a level of exercise that enables you to maintain your pulse at your Target Heart Rate. Maintain this level of exercise, and the peak HR, for 20 minutes. Then slow your pace gradually over 10 minutes to cool down.

Age	Target HR	Maximum Heart Rate
20 years	120 to 150 beats per minute	200
25 years	117 to 146	195
30 years	114 to 142	190
35 years	111 to 138	185
40 years	108 to 135	180
45 years	105 to 131	175
50 years	102 to 127	170
55 years	100 to 123	165
60 years	100 to 120	160
Over 65 years	100 to 115	155

SHOULD YOU LIFT WEIGHTS?

As I've explained, the best exercise for your heart and blood vessels is aerobic. But many people like to lift weights in conjunction with an aerobic fitness program. Is that good for you? It depends on who you are. Lifting heavy weights markedly raises your blood pressure while you are exercising, which is not good for your cardiovascular system. In fact, it is a bad idea for anyone with a heart condition. For people who like to weight train, I recommend reducing the amount of weight you lift. For example, when I bench-press free weights, I lift just 25 pounds, but I do at least 50 repetitions. Or, if I am using Nautilus equipment, I set the weight to the least amount of resistance and do about 50 repetitions. If you can't lift the weight easily 50 times in a row without straining, then you are lifting too much weight and should lift less. (If you are new to weight training, try to lift a light weight 15 times in a row before increasing the number of repetitions.) Lifting light weights, with many repetitions, can help tone the upper-body muscles and is a reasonable exercise, so long as you do many reps without straining.

Getting Started (for Beginners)

YOU WILL need to consult with a physician before you begin exercising, if you

- are at high risk for heart disease
- have heart or vascular disease
- are over the age of 40, haven't been active, and are starting an exercise program for the first time

If you meet any of the criteria above, I recommend a stress test before you embark on an exercise program. In most cases, the stress test is a treadmill study in which you walk (or jog) on a treadmill while attached to an EKG. The physician will determine if there are any worrisome EKG changes consistent with significant coronary artery disease. This test will determine how far you can safely push yourself. After the test, your doctor should be able to give you a Target Heart Rate that you should not exceed during exercise. I watch my patients very carefully when they are on the treadmill; in this way, I can determine the heart rate at which they develop symptoms or changes in their EKG. After the treadmill test, the Target Heart Rate I give them for their exercise program is about 15 beats per minute below the heart rate at which they developed symptoms or EKG changes. During exercise, these patients should not get their heart rate above the target. I show them how to monitor their heart rate (by taking the pulse) or have them invest in a heart rate monitor. These devices are relatively inexpensive and can be purchased in most pharmacies.

Once your doctor gives you the go-ahead to start an exercise program, you can begin. Many people start off a new exercise with great enthusiasm, only to lose steam soon afterward.

Here are some ways to introduce regular exercise into your life:

1. Start slowly. The best way to start an exercise program (and stick with it) is to start slowly. What do I mean by this? Try to fit in short periods of physical activity, so that the idea of physical activity doesn't loom large or seem overwhelming. Don't set your expectations too high. If you create too big a challenge for yourself—or set too large a goal—you simply won't be able to achieve it and you'll get discouraged.

2. Look for opportunities. Take advantage of opportunities throughout the day to increase the amount of physical activity you do. Don't take the elevator; walk up the stairs. Hauling groceries, walking to the mailbox, and weeding are examples of simple activities that you can do around the house. Make the most of these. If you have been sedentary, then catching five minutes of increased activity here or there will add up. What you are doing is not as important as that you are doing something. Moving around a little bit is better than not moving around at all.

For example, try to get 10 or 15 minutes of walking into your daily schedule. Take a walk at lunch or park your car a little farther away from the store in the parking lot so that you have to walk a little farther. Once you are comfortable walking for 10 or 15 minutes, add a few more minutes.

3. Do something you enjoy. Think about activities that you like. Do you like the water? Go for a swim, row a boat, or wade in the water. Is there an exercise class that you'd like to join? Dancing is a good way to get exercise. It doesn't matter what you do, so long as the exercise is aerobic and you do it regularly.

Starting a Walking Program for the First Time

WHY WALK? It's simple. Because it's the easiest, most natural thing to do. All you need are comfortable clothes, the right shoes (see below), and the great outdoors (or indoors—mall walk during the cold winter months).

Walking does wonders for your body. It feels good, it can be social (go for a walk with a friend and see how fast the time goes), it's good for your heart and your health, and it burns calories.

Suiting up. Wear loose, comfortable, weather-appropriate clothing. Most likely, you will warm up once you get started, so don't overdress.

Footwear is especially important. Don't walk in just any shoes; you could hurt your feet. There are athletic shoes or sneakers designed especially for walking; they have a wedge-shaped heel to cushion your landing. Make sure that they fit right; walking shoes should be a little longer than your foot, with a finger's width between your biggest toe and the top of the shoe.

Planning your route. Like any exercise program, you'll want to start small and build. As explained above, plan an easy 10- or 15-minute walk around the block or down a quiet road. (If you have been sedentary and are just starting a walking program, remember that the amount of time that you walk is not as important as that you do it. Once you get used to walking for 10 minutes, add 3 more minutes to your route—and so on, until you can walk for 30 minutes comfortably.) Choose any location that appeals to you: a parking lot, mall, walking path, the sidewalks in your neighborhood, or a local park.

Warming up. The best way to get your body ready for physical exercise is to start slowly. You might have heard that the best way to warm up the body is to stretch your muscles before beginning physical activity. But muscles perform better when they're warmed up. You wouldn't want to stretch your muscles before they're warmed up—that's how you risk injury.

So begin your physical activity by simply doing the activity slowly. If you are planning a 30-minute walk, start by walking slowly for about 5 minutes. You may feel slightly warm, the sign that your muscles have warmed up and are ready to pick up the pace.

Working out. Once you are warmed up and have picked up the pace, increase your walking speed to one that will make you sweat, but that you will be able to maintain for about 20 minutes. Your breathing rate should increase slightly; if you are walking with a friend, it should become a little more difficult to talk as you walk. Your goal should be to increase your heart rate to the peak heart rate as determined from the Target Heart Rate table on p. 170 and maintain that heart rate for about 20 minutes. If you are on medicine to slow down your heart rate, you should ask your doctor about the optimum heart rate for you while walking briskly. As noted above, a supervised treadmill test can help your physician determine your peak heart rate during exercise.

Cooling down. The cool-down should last for about 10 minutes. Like the warm-up, the cool-down helps your body go from being active to returning to normal. About 10 minutes before you end your walk, begin to slow down. You don't want to go from a full-stride, quick-pace movement to no activity at all—stopping abruptly may actually be a strain on your heart and vessels. Instead, by slowing down your pace to a comfortable level (and letting your breathing and heart rate return to normal), you are giving your whole body a chance to comfortably return to its normal state.

Improving Your Fitness as a Walker

ONCE YOU'VE started your walking program, it's important to continue it. There are a number of ways that you can vary or improve your fitness as a walker.

Add variety by varying your routine. For example, pick up the walking pace for 5 minutes, then return to your usual pace for the rest of the walk. Try the quicker pace a few times. When it becomes easier for you, walk at your normal pace for 5 minutes, fast for 5, then normal, then fast again. When you really feel comfortable at the faster pace, pick up the pace for your whole walk. You might also want to try to do your route faster; for example, do your regular 30-minute walk in a couple of minutes less.

Challenge yourself by walking farther. Once your body becomes used to doing a 30-minute walk, try to extend your time (this time, at your normal pace) for 5 more minutes. Once that becomes comfortable, extend it for yet another 5 minutes. Soon you'll be walking longer—and reaping even more benefits.

Staying Motivated

EVEN PEOPLE who exercise regularly must find ways to stay motivated. It isn't easy for anyone. But there are a number of ways to boost your enthusiasm for exercise—the better to keep you going week after week and year after year.

- Challenge yourself. For example, if you like to run or jog but you are becoming bored with your regular routine, think about joining a local race in town. Even if you don't run for speed, you will enjoy the companionship (and the experience). I run in several races during the year; they are challenging and give me something to look forward to and work toward.

- Vary your exercise activities. Find a few activities that you like so that you vary your routine; do an aerobics class one day and swim on another. Doing the same thing over and over again can become boring. Most of the time I run. But I also play tennis with my wife, basketball with my son, and swim with my daughters.

- Branch out. Learn a new activity. Have you always wanted to try the stationary bicycle class called spinning? Go for it. Remember that it might be challenging at first, but the more you do it, the more your body will become used to it.

- Music is a great motivator. Listening to music while you exercise has been shown to keep people working at a greater rate.

- Invest in a personal trainer or join a gym.

- Find an exercise partner. My wife is a member of a walking club; they meet three times a week and walk (and talk) together for an hour. For my part, I lope along with a running club in Palo Alto; with a big group of about 50 people, I can always find someone of equal ability (or better) to help keep the pace. Exercising with people is one way to keep it enjoyable. It's also a way to ensure that you do it. If you don't show up, your exercise partner(s) will want to know why.

- Make an appointment with yourself to exercise. You make an appointment to go to the doctor or dentist. Why not do the same with exercise? If you make an appointment and set aside time to exercise, chances are you will be less willing to break the date with yourself.

- Find the time of day when you feel most energetic. Some people enjoy exercising first thing in the morning, while others choose a time after work.

- Think of exercise as something you do for yourself. Try to do activities that you enjoy. Not only will you be improving your health, but you will feel better for it.

- Go out and play with your kids. That's exercise too.

Remember that the more you do, the more you *can* do. Being healthy, shedding a few pounds, feeling strong and able—these are, after all, some of the very best motivators of all.

USE IT OR LOSE IT?

If you don't use it, you lose it. You may notice that when you stop exercising, your cardiovascular fitness fades. Research has shown that in middle-aged or older people, cardiovascular fitness can decline rapidly, within as little as days to weeks.

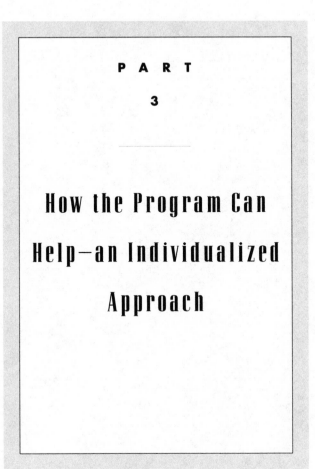

PART

3

How the Program Can Help—an Individualized Approach

Chapter 7

How Healthy Is Your Endothelium?

The executive with diabetes.
The editor with high cholesterol.
The manager with high blood pressure.
The farmer who likes a smoke now and then.
The nurse who is postmenopausal.
The retiree riding the cart around the golf course.

What do these people have in common? You guessed it—these individuals are all at risk for atherosclerosis. But how have they ended up with the same disease, you might ask. They have lost the magic: their endothelium is not healthy and is not producing enough NO. Unfortunately, when you lose the magic of NO, you have taken the first step toward hardening of the arteries—and sustaining a possible heart attack or stroke.

The bad news is that the magic can be lost easily, and lost early. But the good news is that it's never too late to improve your endothelial health.

How Can You Tell if Your Endothelium Is Functioning Normally?

IN THE research laboratory, we have several ways of determining endothelial health. We can measure ADMA levels in the blood. We can measure the metabolites of NO in blood or urine. We can measure expired NO (that's right, as you breathe, you release some NO from your body into the air). We can measure the second messenger of NO (cyclic GMP) in platelets (particles in the blood that form blood clots), blood, or urine. We can measure increases in blood flow in the heart or limb arteries using special equipment. We can also use ultrasound machines to observe increases in the caliber of the arm vessels in response to changes in blood flow.

Unfortunately, these techniques are only available in a few research laboratories and have not been standardized. It will not be long before a test to determine endothelial function will be widely available in the doctor's office. (As this book goes to press, new techniques to measure endothelial function in the doctor's office are becoming available.) In a few years, having your endothelial function tested will be as easy as getting your blood pressure or cholesterol checked—and even more important. In the meantime, how can you assess the health of your endothelium? You could participate as a volunteer in a study involving endothelial health at an academic medical center such as Stanford. Or you can estimate your endothelial function using the system described below.

How Healthy Is Your Endothelium?

YOU KNOW that your endothelium is not healthy if you have any of the symptoms and warning signs of heart disease. (See Chapter 11.) These symptoms are there for a reason; they are your body's way of telling you that your vascular system is in trouble. Let's hope, however, that you don't yet have these signals.

You can estimate your risk of developing heart disease—and know the condition of your endothelium—by assessing your risk factors. In the late 1980s and early 1990s, Drs. Celermajer and Deanfield conducted studies in London to assess endothelial function in hundreds of healthy and not-so-healthy volunteers. Using ultrasound to measure flow-mediated vasodilation (to assess the body's ability to release NO), they found that the number of risk factors correlated with endothelial health: if you had few risk factors, your endothelium was healthy. The greater the number of risk factors, the greater the chance of endothelial health impairment and heart attack.

RISK ASSESSMENT PROFILE

To estimate how well your endothelium is working, take a look at the following risk factors and count how many you have:

1. Tobacco use
2. Diabetes
3. Family history
4. Age (count only if you are a man over 50 or a woman over 60)
5. High cholesterol
6. Hypertension
7. Sedentary lifestyle
8. Obesity

If you have one of these risk factors, it is likely that your endothelium is already showing signs of wear and tear.

If you have two or three risk factors, then you probably have a moderate impairment in endothelial function.

If you have four or five risk factors, your endothelium is probably severely impaired.

If you have more than five risk factors, your endothelium is no longer able to make your vessels relax. Furthermore, you have lost your self-defense against heart attack and stroke.

This assessment gives you a rough idea of your risk of endothelial dysfunction.

If you have any of the risk factors listed above, you need to follow my program to restore and maintain the health of your blood vessels. In the long term, you could avoid a heart attack or stroke, live longer, and feel more vigorous physically and mentally. This is a rough indication of how well your endothelium is functioning. If you want to refine your analysis, use the Point System Risk Assessment, below.

The Point System Risk Assessment

WHAT IS YOUR RISK OF HAVING A HEART ATTACK OR STROKE IN THE NEXT 10 YEARS?

BASED ON decades of research, the American Heart Association and the American College of Cardiology have published a point system to help you determine your risk of developing heart disease over the next 10 years. To estimate your risk, look at Table 1, below. Add up your points based on your age, cholesterol, and blood pressure and whether or not you smoke or have diabetes. Note the number of points you have.

(If you already have symptoms of heart disease, this table is not applicable to you. Your risk of having a heart attack and stroke is high, and you should follow the recommendations in Chapter 11.)

Table 1. The Point System for Assessing Your Risk

Risk Factor	Risk Points (Men)	Risk Points (Women)
Age		
<34	-1	-9
35–39	0	-4
40–44	1	0
45–49	2	3
50–54	3	6
55–59	4	7
60–64	5	8
65–69	6	8
70–74	7	8
Total cholesterol (mg/dl)		
<160	-3	-2
169–199	0	0
200–239	1	1
240–279	2	2
>280	3	3
HDL cholesterol (mg/dl)		
<35	2	5
35–44	1	2
45–49	0	1

50–59	0	0
>60	-2	-3

Systolic blood pressure (mmHg)

<120	0	-3
120–129	0	0
130–139	1	1
140–159	2	2
160	3	3

Diabetes (fasting blood sugar >126)

No	0	0
Yes	2	4

Smoker

No	0	0
Yes	2	2

Using the number of points added together in Table 1, use Table 2 (see p. 184) to figure out your risk of having a heart problem over the next 10 years.

TAKING INTO ACCOUNT OTHER FACTORS

ALTHOUGH THIS table provides you with a rough idea of your risk, it does not take into account all of the risk factors, such as ethnicity, or the magnitude of certain risk factors, such as the severity of your diabetes or amount of your tobacco use. For a more accurate reading, consider the following factors and adjust your score accordingly.

Ethnicity
If you are East Asian (Japanese), the table may overestimate your risk by about 30 percent. To get a better estimate, multiply your points by 0.67.

If you are South Asian (Indian or Pakistani) but living in a Western society (and eating a Western diet), your risk of heart disease is underestimated by the table. To get a better estimate, multiple your points by 2.

Adjusting for Other Factors

· If you are a heavy smoker (more than one pack a day), add 1 point.

- If your diabetes is not well controlled (a fasting blood sugar greater than 150 or a glycosylated hemoglobin greater than 8), add 1 point.

- If you are sedentary (you exercise fewer than three times a week), add 1 point.

- If you exercise regularly (walk, jog, swim, bike, or take an aerobics class for 30 minutes at least five times a week), subtract 1 point.

- If you are obese (more than 20 percent overweight or more than 30 kg/m^2), add 1 point.

- Even with these adjustments, the table is not perfect. It does not take into account a family history of premature heart disease. If someone in your family has had symptoms of hardening of the arteries at a young age (under the age of 55), your risk is further increased; add 2 points.

- If you are a woman under the age of 50 but have already reached menopause, add 2 points.

Table 2. Calculating Your Risk of a Heart Attack or Stroke in the Next 10 Years

Points	Your Risk (Men)	Your Risk (Women)
0	2%	2%
1	3	2
2	4	3
3	5	3
4	7	4
5	8	4
6	10	5
7	13	6
8	16	7
9	20	8
10	25	10
11	31	11
12	37	13
13	45	15
14	>50	18
15	>50	20

| 16 | >50 | 24 |
| 17 | >50 | 27 |

Add up your points and find out your risk for developing heart disease over the next 10 years. Your score will determine which chapter you need to focus on at the end of this book.

For men:

If your score is 3 or below, you are in good shape. You will want to maintain your vascular health on into the future. To do this, read Chapter 8, The Worried Well—Maintaining the Health of the Endothelium.

If your score is 4 to 6, your endothelium is moderately impaired, and you are at risk of developing heart disease. Follow the recommendations in Chapter 9, Reducing Risk—Repairing and Restoring the Endothelium.

If your score is 6 to 10, your endothelium is probably severely impaired. Over the course of your lifetime, your risk for having a heart attack is dangerously high. Follow the recommendations in Chapter 11, Already Ill—Intensive Care for Your Blood Vessels.

If your score is over 10, your endothelium is in bad shape, and it is likely that you already have a significant amount of plaque in your vessels. In either case, it is time for you to follow the recommendations in Chapter 11, Already Ill—Intensive Care for Your Blood Vessels.

For women:

If your score is 5 or below, you are in good shape. You will want to maintain your vascular health on into the future. To do this, read Chapter 8, The Worried Well—Maintaining the Health of the Endothelium.

If your score is 6 to 10, your endothelium is moderately impaired, and you are at risk of developing heart disease. Follow the recommendations in Chapter 9, Reducing Risk—Repairing and Restoring the Endothelium.

If your score is 11 to 15, your endothelium is probably severely impaired. Over the course of your lifetime, your risk for having a heart attack is dangerously high. Follow the recommendations in Chapter 11, Already Ill—Intensive Care for Your Blood Vessels.

If your score is over 15, your endothelium is in bad shape, and it is likely that you already have a significant amount of plaque in your vessels. In either case, it is time for you to follow the recommendations in Chapter 11, Already Ill—Intensive Care for Your Blood Vessels.

WHAT IS YOUR RISK BASED ON AGE AND GENDER?

The risk of having a heart attack or stroke is much too high for the average American. For example, note that a 60-year-old man has a one-in-five chance of having a heart attack or stroke over the next 10 years. This table assesses the average risk for developing hardening of the arteries over the next 10 years.

Age	Average Risk (Man)	Average Risk (Woman)
30–34	3%	2%
35–39	5	2
40–44	7	5
45–49	10	6
50–54	13	8
55–59	16	10
60–64	20	11
65–69	25	13
70–74	31	15

Source: Framingham Heart Study

Chapter 8

The Worried Well—
Maintaining the Health of
the Endothelium

The advice in this chapter applies to men who scored less than 3 or women who scored less than 5 on The Point System Risk Assessment in Chapter 7. At this point, your blood vessels are healthy. You are concerned, though, about maintaining your cardiovascular health in the future.

There are a number of things you can do to ensure your vascular health. You can continue to stay healthy, and ensure your future cardiovascular health, by doing the following:

- Stick with my diet, since it is especially designed to enhance vascular health.

- Continue to maintain a healthy weight. My diet will help you do this. When you are a healthy weight for your size and frame, you make it easier for the endothelium to do its job. The endothelium can pump NO as it needs to, without interference from high blood levels of cholesterol, triglycerides, or blood sugar.

- Continue, or start, an exercise program. My recommendation is to perform vigorous activity for at least 30 minutes, at least four days a week.

- Monitor your health by having regular checkups with your physician.

How You'll Benefit from a Vigorous Exercise Program

FOR HEART and blood vessel health, the best type of exercise is aerobic. Since you are someone who is fairly healthy and at low risk for heart disease, you should be able to build up to a program of vigorous exercise (swimming, jogging, biking, or walking) for at least 30 minutes, at least four days a week.

After you have been exercising regularly for a few weeks, your heart rate at rest will begin to decrease, as will your blood pressure. Over a few weeks to months, your LDL (bad) cholesterol will decrease and your HDL (good) cholesterol will increase. In addition, over a few months your body will become more responsive to the insulin that it makes, and your blood sugar and triglycerides will fall to lower levels. Your energy and alertness will be enhanced, and you will sleep well at night.

Regular exercise will also strengthen your blood vessels. They will make more NO and less oxygen-derived free radicals. The antioxidant self-defense system in your blood vessels will be maximally activated. As a result, oxidative stress in your blood vessels will be markedly reduced. Remember that these free radicals are agents of destruction, and they accelerate the aging process. By reducing these free radicals and strengthening your body's antioxidant defense mechanism, you will slow down, and even reverse, the aging process.

Designing Your Workout

TO GET the most benefit from a 30-minute workout, set it up with the following in mind:

- 5-minute warm-up. If you are running, start slowly and let your body warm up for about 5 minutes. Throughout the 5 minutes, gradually increase your pace.

- The workout. Sustain the increased pace for 20 minutes of continuous and strenuous exertion at 50 to 75 percent of your maximum heart rate. (See the Target Heart Rate table in Chapter 6.)

- 5-minute cool-down. If you are jogging, slow your pace over a period of 5 minutes until you are walking.

Should you do more? There is evidence that participating in more prolonged and vigorous activity can further improve your cardiovascular system. But avoid intermittent bouts of extreme exertion, otherwise known as the weekend-athlete syndrome. It is much better to exercise at a consistent moderate or vigorous level and maintain that level of physical activity year in and year out.

IF YOU ARE HEALTHY BUT DON'T EXERCISE, TRY TO START AN EXERCISE PROGRAM

Remember that even a small amount of physical activity can help lower the risk of cardiovascular disease. Try to do some type of physical activity every day. Gradually increase your exercise time until you can participate in moderate- or low-intensity aerobic activity. (See Chapter 6 for more information on getting started.)

Chapter 9

Reducing Risk—
Repairing and Restoring the Endothelium

T HE ADVICE in this chapter applies to men who scored 4 to 6 or women who scored 6 to 10 on the Point System Risk Assessment in Chapter 7. You have elevated levels of ADMA, your endothelium is moderately impaired, and you are at risk of developing heart disease. You may have vessel disease already, but you don't have any symptoms. It is now time to restore your endothelial health and reduce your risk factors before serious damage is done.

What can you do about this? Plenty. You are never too old or too unhealthy to reverse the damage of atherosclerosis.

The first steps you must take:

- Follow my diet.
- Begin or continue an exercise program.
- Reduce your risk factors (see below).

Your blood vessels are living tissues that are exquisitely sensitive to what you do. When healthy, they are flexible and can relax with increases in blood flow. But if you eat one high-fat meal, your blood vessels don't dilate as well. If you smoke one cigarette, your blood vessels constrict. If your blood vessels take this abuse over the course of many years, they respond by becoming stiff and thick. But blood vessels will respond to a healthy lifestyle—including diet, exercise, and supplements—and a reduction in risk factors.

Here's how to start undoing the damage and repairing the endothelium by reducing your risk factors.

Tobacco Use

ALTHOUGH IT is well known that tobacco use puts you at grave risk for developing lung cancer and emphysema, smoking causes more deaths because of the damage it causes to blood vessels and the rate at which it accelerates atherosclerosis.

So far, researchers know that carbon monoxide and cadmium cause some of the damage. Nitric oxide takes a big hit. The free radicals in smoke reduce nitric oxide in the blood vessels and cause an increase in ADMA. This creates a vicious cycle in which the vessels can't make more NO to make up for the amount that was destroyed.

The tars and nitrosamines in smoke can make tissues grow abnormally and may cause cancer. My laboratory at Stanford has recently shown that nicotine in cigarettes can cause blood vessels to grow tumors, nourishing them and increasing their growth.

Nicotine can also accelerate the growth of plaque that can clog your heart, brain, leg, and abdominal vessels. How does this happen? Plaque may look inanimate, but it is full of living cells that need nourishment to grow. These cells make substances that cause tiny threads of blood vessels to grow into the plaque in a process known as neovascularization (the creation of new vessels). Nicotine accelerates the growth of these little threads of vessels, nourishing the plaque and ensuring that it continues to grow in the vessel wall, just like a tumor grows.

When you smoke, you also cause some immediate changes in the body that strain the heart. Blood pressure and heart rate increase. Arteries narrow. Blood is less able to deliver oxygen to the heart. Platelets become stickier and can more easily form a clot. Even passive smoking (exposure to the cigarette smoke of someone else) takes its toll, causing the same damage as smoking itself, as documented by Dr. William Parmley and colleagues at UCSF.

Reducing the risk: The answer to reducing this risk is obvious. Quit smoking. Obviously, that's easier said than done. Nicotine addiction is one of the hardest addictions to break. But it can be done. A multicenter study led by researchers at the Mayo Clinic Nicotine Dependence Center found that men are generally more successful at stopping smoking than women, and that the first two weeks of abstinence is the most critical in predicting long-term cessation success.

Your physician may recommend nicotine gum or patches that can help, if used correctly. By all means, take advantage of these helpful tools. But remember that gum and patches should only be used for a few weeks. Short-term use is safe. Prolonged use of nicotine gum and patches could be harmful and should be avoided. (By the way, it is not advisable to use nicotine gum or patches to help lose weight.) There are other helpful medications that can increase your chances of successfully kicking the habit. Ask your doctor about clonidine and bupropion, drugs that help the brain reduce craving. The combination of bupropion with nicotine patch treatment is more successful than either one alone, as shown by a randomized clinical trial.

There are many community-based smoking cessation groups. They take advantage of new techniques in behavioral therapy that can help people stop smoking or avoid falling back into the habit. Check your local YMCA or hospital. Or ask your physician to recommend a cessation program in your area.

Diabetes

TODAY, THERE is alarming news about diabetes, already known as the "silent epidemic," affecting about 16 million Americans. It used to be that the most common type of diabetes—Type 2 or adult-onset—affected just adults. But the Centers for Disease Control and Prevention now report that the age at which Type 2 strikes (it was in middle age or older) is decreasing and affecting more young adults and teenagers than ever before. This increase in diabetes is due to the epidemic of obesity and the increase of refined carbohydrates in the diet. Diabetes is a disorder in which the body is unable to metabolize glucose, the sugar molecule that is carried in the blood and used to fuel the body. Normally, blood sugar, or glucose, as it is called, is regulated by the hormone insulin. Insulin, secreted in response to a rise in blood sugar, prepares the receptors on muscle cells to absorb the glucose. In a normal blood vessel, the glucose is absorbed and used by the muscle cells, and then the blood sugar returns to normal. In Type 1 diabetes, people have a shortage of insulin—and need insulin injections in order to prepare the cells to do their job. Without the insulin, their cells would not function normally.

By contrast, people with Type 2, or adult-onset, diabetes can produce insulin. But their bodies no longer respond to the insulin they do make. For a while, their bodies attempt to make more insulin to make up for the resistance. But after a while, their production of insulin cannot keep up with the increased resistance to insulin—and blood sugar rises. The initial treatment is weight loss and the right diet, like mine, which helps maintain or lose weight, thus lowering blood sugar levels. Medication or insulin injections may also be required.

In addition, people with Type 2 diabetes often have high blood pressure. A recent study from England shows that in people with diabetes, controlling blood pressure is even more important than controlling blood sugar! In people with diabetes, blood pressure should be about 120/80 mmHg. Even a modest elevation over this level can increase the risk of heart attack or stroke. For many patients, diet and exercise do not decrease high blood pressure, and patients often need medication.

The majority of patients with diabetes also have abnormal blood lipids. Typically, the good (HDL) cholesterol is too low, and the triglycerides in the blood are too high. The bad (LDL) cholesterol may be in a normal range (although even normal levels of LDL cholesterol may be too high for a person with diabetes). If these blood lipid abnormalities are not corrected with diet and exercise, then cholesterol-lowering medicine may be necessary.

People who have diabetes tend to get a particularly bad form of atherosclerosis because it tends to affect the smaller, as well as larger, vessels. If these patients have angina or leg pain that is unresponsive to medication, it is often difficult to correct their problem with surgery or angioplasty because the whole vascular tree (both large and smaller vessels going to the heart and limbs) are affected. People with diabetes also get an unusual overgrowth of tiny vessels in their eyes that can cause blindness if these fragile eye vessels rupture and bleed. These patients also have kidney and nerve disease related to small vessel disease and endothelial dysfunction.

Reducing the risk: My diet is especially geared to controlling blood sugar and reducing the progression of vascular disease. By following it, you can reduce your chance of developing diabetes and reduce the complications of vascular disease if you already have diabetes. We know that in people with diabetes, the endothelium makes too much superoxide anion and destroys NO. In these individuals, an oral dose of vitamin C (2 grams) can improve flow-mediated vasodilation in the short term. In the long run, it is far better to simply have seven to nine helpings of fruit and vegetables every day—and get an abundant supply of antioxidants that way. (People with diabetes should eat whole fruits and avoid fruit juices. Whole fruits contain fiber that slows down the absorption of sugar in the fruit.) Vascular problems related to diabetes can be prevented or delayed with aggressive control of blood sugar, blood pressure, and blood lipids, using a combination of diet, supplements and vitamins, exercise, and the right medications. As for the latter, there are now more medications than ever to help patients control their blood sugar, including drugs with different forms of insulin; drugs that can make the body more sensitive to its own insulin; and drugs that can increase the insulin released from the pancreas. If you have diabetes, you need to see an endocrinologist or an internist specializing in diabetes, who can tailor medications to your needs. If you follow the diet and exercise recommendations in this book, it is likely that you will need less medication in the future.

Family History

THERE IS some unique characteristic in your genetic makeup that predisposes you to hardening of the arteries. Some of these hereditary risk factors have been identified, and your doctor should test for them if you have a family history of premature heart attack or stroke.

One of these hereditary risk factors is lipoprotein (a). Lipoprotein (a)—also known as Lp(a)—is a substance similar to, but worse than, LDL (bad) cholesterol. Lp(a) is stickier and more likely to accelerate blood clot and plaque formation.

Another hereditary risk factor is high blood levels of homocysteine, the modified amino acid that damages blood vessels and accelerates atherosclerosis. Fortunately, the severe form of this genetic disorder is rare in children and young adults. However, even slight elevations in homocysteine levels can accelerate hardening of the arteries. As it turns out, slight elevations of homocysteine are common.

If you have blood levels of homocysteine greater than 12 (the normal range is 6 to 10), your endothelium is not healthy, and you are more likely to develop hardening of the arteries. The Physicians' Health Study showed that people with high homocysteine levels were three times more likely to have a heart attack over a five-year period. Homocysteine levels are often too high in people who have kidney or liver impairment, in people who have some genetic disorders, and in people who are deficient in B vitamins. The latter is the most common cause of elevated homocysteine levels. Folate helps to convert homocysteine back into methionine, and B$_6$ helps change homocysteine into a substance that can be excreted in the urine.

Reducing the risk: If you have a family history of premature hardening of the arteries, you should be tested for high levels of homocysteine and lipoprotein (a), because the treatment for these risk factors—the addition of B vitamins to treat high homocysteine; and niacin, fish oil, and/or estrogen to reduce Lp(a)—is somewhat different from treatment for the other risk factors.

Lipoprotein (a) is a particularly harmful factor that can't be reduced by statins. Nevertheless, statins are useful for people with high levels of lipoprotein (a) because they are very good at reducing LDL cholesterol, and it is best to have a lower LDL cholesterol level if you have high Lp(a). Because it is such a strong risk factor for heart disease, it is also important to try to reduce high levels of lipoprotein (a) with fish oil and niacin (see Chapter 10 for a discussion of these helpful supplements).

Age (50+ Years for a Man; 60+ Years for a Woman)

UNDER THE age of 65, men are at greater risk from heart attack and stroke than women. Women appear to be protected from heart attack and stroke until they go through menopause. Accordingly, there is about a 10-year lag before women begin to succumb to vascular problems. This has led to the false impression that women do not have as much problem with heart attack and stroke. Nothing could be further from the truth. After menopause, women begin to catch up to men in terms of heart disease. As it turns out, the major cause of death in women is not breast, ovarian, or uterine cancer; it is heart attack and stroke. In fact, the unfortunate woman who has a heart attack at an early age (around 50) is more likely to die during this event than a man of the same age.

Why are premenopausal women protected from these risk factors? The most likely cause is the hormonal difference between men and women. Estrogen, in particular, has many benefits, including the ability to increase the expression of NO synthase, the enzyme that makes NO. Accordingly, premenopausal women make more NO than men of the same age. As women enter menopause, they lose this advantage. The endothelial function of postmenopausal women is no different from that of men in the same age group.

Reducing the risk: Research has shown that estrogens from plants, phytoestrogens, can help protect the body from cardiovascular disease. Men and women who consume more soy protein have fewer heart attacks and strokes. In addition, soy can reduce hot flashes in women who are going through menopause.

Because two recent large randomized clinical trials (HERS and ERA) showed that estrogen did not reduce heart attack and stroke in at-risk postmenopausal women, I no longer recommend the use of estrogen for prevention of heart disease in all women. However, in selected cases, I do recommend estrogen. In postmenopausal women who have high Lp(a), estrogen may help reduce the Lp(a) level. Estrogen replacement is also a good therapy for postmenopausal women at great risk of osteoporosis or for those who have severe menopausal symptoms (hot flashes) that are not responsive to soy or soy supplements.

High Cholesterol

SINCE THE 1960s, researchers have known about the link between cholesterol and atherosclerosis. And many studies have shown that lowering cholesterol can reduce the risk of heart attack or stroke. We know that

- If you have cholesterol over 200, you are at increased risk of heart attack or stroke.

- If your cholesterol is greater than 200, you need a lipid profile to determine your levels of bad (LDL) and good (HDL) cholesterol.

• An LDL cholesterol of 160 or greater puts you at risk even if you are young. (If you are over the age of 45 years, even an LDL cholesterol over 100 puts you at somewhat greater risk; if you want to be at the lowest risk, get your LDL cholesterol under 100.)

• An HDL cholesterol of 45 or less also puts you at risk.

• An HDL cholesterol of 60 or greater *significantly* reduces your risk.

(A word of caution: elevated levels of LDL cholesterol put you at risk for heart attack and stroke—and senility. That's because after Alzheimer's disease, the most common cause of dementia is vascular disease. Multiple small strokes can rob you of your intellect and personality. In a study of over 1,000 healthy elderly people in New York City during a two-year period, researchers found that a high LDL cholesterol caused a fourfold risk of vascular dementia.)

Reducing the risk: We now know much more about cholesterol and its role in heart attack and stroke, and we have better medications to reduce cholesterol. Statins have revolutionized our ability to reduce cholesterol and to reduce heart attack and stroke. Statins also improve NO production and blood flow by increasing the activity of NO synthase in the vessel wall and reducing the amount of free radicals produced there.

In patients with coronary artery disease and high blood cholesterol at the Brigham and Women's Cardiac Catheterization Laboratory, an aggressive lipid-lowering regimen with a statin improved endothelial function in the coronary arteries after six months. Statins improve endothelial function in several ways. First, high levels of cholesterol cause the vessel to make free radicals that destroy NO. Reduce cholesterol level and you reduce a stimulus for the production of free radicals. Second, free radicals reduce the activity of DDAH, and thereby increase ADMA (the molecule that blocks NO production). Finally, statins cause the vessel to make more NO synthase.

If you have high cholesterol but are young and otherwise healthy, you can probably get your cholesterol to safe levels following my diet and exercise program. I also recommend niacin as a safe nutritional supplement for lowering cholesterol. The sterol- or stanol-containing margarine substitutes can also reduce cholesterol by about 10 to

15 percent. In addition, garlic, fish oil, and policosanol (a supplement that is a waxy substance derived from sugarcane) can also be effective nutritional therapies to lower cholesterol levels. (For more information about these dietary supplements, see Chapter 10.) However, if these natural strategies don't get your cholesterol into a safe range, and if you have other risk factors, you need medication.

THE COMPLEXITIES OF LOWERING CHOLESTEROL

Because everyone is different, my goal in lowering cholesterol depends on each individual's risk.

• If you have high cholesterol but are young and otherwise healthy, I would like your total cholesterol to be under 200 mg/dl and your LDL (bad) cholesterol under 160 mg/dl, and preferably under 130. If your cholesterol is higher than this, I recommend that you have your cholesterol checked after eight weeks of following my diet. If it remains high, it is time to try lipid-lowering supplements (see Chapter 10) to see if these can lower your cholesterol.

• If you have high cholesterol and multiple risk factors for vessel disease (family history, tobacco use, hypertension, diabetes mellitus), you should see a doctor who can guide you in the selection of supplements or the initiation of medication. I would recommend my diet and medication and/or supplementation, started simultaneously. Most people get, at most, a 10 percent reduction in total cholesterol from diet. But if you have multiple risk factors (or symptoms of heart disease), it is hard to get LDL cholesterol under 100 mg/dl with diet and nutritional supplements alone. For such people I would first recommend a statin. Other cholesterol-lowering medicines that are useful include cholesterol-binding resins and high-dose niacin (with doses slowly increasing over time up to 2 grams). This aggressive approach to LDL cholesterol in people who are already suffering from heart disease is justified by large clinical studies showing the benefits in these very-high-risk people. For example, the NHLBI Post Coronary Artery Bypass Graft Clinical Trial demonstrated that lowering LDL cholesterol to under 100 reduced blockages in bypass grafts by over 30 percent in comparison to people who had LDL cholesterol reduced to only 130. There are at least two dozen trials with statins showing that aggressive lowering of cholesterol can slow the progression of atherosclerosis and reduce your risk of heart attack and stroke by about 25 percent.

• The focus of the medical community is on reducing the LDL (bad) cholesterol, and for good reason, since elevated levels of LDL cholesterol correlate better with heart disease than do other lipid fractions. However, the amount of HDL (good) cholesterol is also important. There is less agreement on what constitutes a healthy HDL cholesterol, level, but levels under 50 mg/dl are not healthy, and levels under 45 mg/dl definitely put you at risk for heart disease. There are a number of things that you can do to naturally increase your HDL cholesterol (such as exercising daily and drinking one or two glasses of red wine or an alcohol beverage daily). However, if you are at higher risk as described above, and your HDL cholesterol levels have not increased with the natural methods discussed, you may need medication.

Hypertension or High Blood Pressure

THIS DISORDER is an excessive pressure of the blood against the walls of the vessels and heart. It is one of the most common ailments in the U.S., the most frequent cause of stroke, and one of the major risk factors for heart disease. Also known as the "silent killer," hypertension often causes no symptoms, but instead gradually damages the heart, vessels, tissues, and organs.

Blood pressure varies minute by minute depending on what you are doing: reading, jogging, sleeping. When you are asleep, blood pressure is at its lowest point, and it increases as you awaken in the morning. The normal blood pressure ranges from 100 to 140 mmHg systolic (the upper number) and 60 to 80 diastolic (the lower number).

High blood pressure (hypertension) increases your risk of having a heart attack or stroke. The systolic number is a particularly important predictor of your risk for stroke. A systolic pressure greater than 150 mmHg increases your risk.

Over time, hypertension damages your blood vessels. The vessel coat begins to thicken and the overlying endothelium becomes sticky. NO activity becomes impaired, increasing blood pressure even further (by reducing the ability of the blood vessels to relax). All of these processes accelerate hardening of the arteries.

Hypertension also wears out your heart. Initially, the heart walls thicken in response to the strain of working against the increased pressure. But then the heart doesn't contract as forcefully. As this condition worsens, heart failure develops. Hypertension is the most common cause of heart failure in this country.

Reducing the risk: People with high blood pressure or advanced hypertension typically have a severe deficiency of NO synthase in the vessel wall. These patients need a combined program, including my diet and exercise program, nutritional supplements, and medication. (I discuss the best medicines to reduce blood pressure in Chapter 11.)

Sedentary State

PEOPLE WHO are sedentary are twice as likely to succumb to a heart attack or stroke than people who are active. Just think about it: if you don't move around, you don't get your blood vessels revved up and functioning at peak levels. Daily exercise reduces many risk factors, including LDL (bad) cholesterol (while increasing HDL [good] cholesterol), blood sugar, stress hormones (such as adrenaline), resting heart rate and blood pressure, and weight. Exercise also directly benefits your endothelium.

Reducing the risk: You don't have to be an ultramarathoner to benefit from exercise; even moderate daily exertion (vigorous walking for 30 minutes daily) can add years to your life. (See my recommendations for exercise in Chapter 6.)

Obesity

MORE AND more Americans are obese. One of the reasons for this rise might be misleading dietary guidelines in the past few years. Many Americans have reduced their saturated fat intake (a good thing), but replaced that fat with refined carbohydrates (not a good thing). Two-thirds of my heart disease patients have high triglycerides and low HDL cholesterol, problems made worse by eating too many refined carbohydrates. These individuals are overweight and often have high blood pressure. People with these risk factors (high triglycerides, low HDL cholesterol, high blood pressure, and obesity) often have a syndrome called insulin resistance, which means that they need to make much more insulin to keep their blood sugar in the normal range. Ultra-low-fat diets often make these individuals worse. A moderate intake of "good" fats and use of complex whole grain carbohydrates and plant-based protein (as in my diet) is the perfect nutrition for these individuals.

To summarize, obesity brings with it a host of health problems, including high glucose and insulin resistance, high triglycerides, and lower HDL (good) cholesterol—all factors that damage the endothelium.

Reducing the risk: Work on maintaining a healthy weight. Shedding even a few pounds can start you on your way to a healthier heart and blood vessels. My diet will help you gradually reduce your weight; in addition, the diet increases intake of healthy fats and nutrient-rich carbohydrates found in fruit, vegetables, nuts, beans, and legumes.

Stress

STRESS TAKES its toll on the blood vessels. Like other muscles in the body, blood vessels contract and expand in response to the nervous system. Nerves from the subconscious depths of our brain extend to the spinal cord and branch out as nerve fibers in the blood vessels. Fear, anxiety, and stress can activate the nerve fibers of our blood vessels, releasing adrenaline-like substances into the vessel wall, causing it to relax or constrict. This explains how emotion can trigger angina, when individuals have blood vessels narrowed by plaque. The emotional stress activates the nerves in the blood vessels, causing them to constrict.

The vasoconstrictor nerves that are activated by anger or other strong emotions also stimulate the adrenal gland to release adrenaline into the bloodstream. Adrenaline makes the heart race. It also constricts vessels in the skin and gut and relaxes vessels to the heart and brain (to redirect blood to where it's needed in a fight-or-flight situation). Adrenaline also enhances the ability of the blood to clot. From an evolutionary standpoint, these are appropriate physiological reactions if you have encountered a saber-toothed tiger, but not if you are caught in a traffic jam.

There are other nerves that slow the heartbeat and cause blood vessels to relax and open. Obviously, if you had a choice, you would prefer that these nerves have a greater influence on your coronary arteries and heart. The goal behind stress reduction is to do just that, tip the balance in favor of these parasympathetic nerves that cause vessel relaxation.

Reducing the risk: Many types of gentle exercise techniques, such as yoga, have been shown to reduce stress and relax both mind and body. Some people find that it helps to turn to a spiritual adviser, family counselor, or psychologist. There are many paths to inner tranquillity. The particular path you choose is not as important as the destination.

FOR MORE INFORMATION . . .

For more information on starting an exercise program, see Chapter 6.

For more information on supplements, see Chapter 10.

For more information on medications, see Chapter 11.

Chapter 10

Dietary Supplements for Heart Health

VER THE last few years, we have been deluged by advertisements and promotions for vitamins and herbal products that claim to do all kinds of things—make us feel more vigorous, lose weight, enhance our sex life, improve mental function, and, yes, even reduce symptoms of heart disease. Are these claims accurate? Are the products safe? Should we take them?

As with anything, there are pros and cons to taking dietary supplements. (By dietary supplements, I mean vitamins, amino acids, minerals, and herbal extracts.) Dietary supplements have not all been rigorously tested; they are not all of the same quality; and the claims for some products are not substantiated. (For details, see The Booming Health Food Industry, p. 204.)

Nevertheless, there are some useful supplements available to help the heart and blood vessels. In general, nutritional supplements tend to be milder than drugs in their actions and their side effects. For example, in clinical trials, ginkgo biloba increases walking distance on a treadmill in patients with peripheral arterial disease. But it doesn't increase walking distance as effectively as the drug cilostazol, which improves walking distance by about 50 percent. (Cilostazol is a drug that can help reduce leg pain due to blockages in the blood vessels there.) On the other hand, ginkgo is easier on your body than cilostazol, which is also known to increase heart rate and can cause palpitations and headache.

As a physician/scientist, I base my recommendations for the use of dietary supplements on the clinical research that does exist about them. Before making any recommendation, I determine if any studies substantiate their use. Therefore, you can be sure that each supplement that I recommend has been clinically tested (although in general the clinical trials of supplements tend to be smaller than those for a medication).

In this chapter, you will find out about these alternative treatments and whether they will work for you. Realize that these vitamins and herbal products will not replace a healthy diet and exercise. It is also important to understand that each individual is different and that supplements work differently for each person, as do medications. You and your doctor should seek to find the combination of supplements—and, if need be, medications—that works for you.

THE BOOMING HEALTH FOOD INDUSTRY

Despite concerns about health food products, it is a booming business. In fact, about 40 percent of all Americans use some form of dietary supplement. Vitamins lead the list in terms of numbers and total spent on sales, followed by botanicals.[1] It is estimated that 50 percent of the American public has used alternative therapies including dietary supplements.[2] In my opinion, there is an overutilization of supplements by the American public and, by contrast, underutilization of these natural therapies by American physicians. Nutritional therapies and supplements have traditionally been overlooked by physicians in the U.S., largely because of the perception (somewhat justified) that the health food field lacks scientific rigor and is not well regulated.

For the pharmaceutical companies, developing new medications is a risky and expensive business. Before receiving FDA approval, a new drug goes through many years of animal testing and human studies, costing several hundred million dollars. The FDA also makes rigorous demands on pharmaceutical companies for quality control of manufacturing, marketing, and distribution. The end product of these stringent controls is usually a drug that is of high quality and efficacy, but that is also expensive.

By contrast, health food companies are not required to perform research on their products, and quality control is minimal. (In 1994, Congress passed the Dietary Supplement Health and Education Act [DSHEA], which permits the health food industry to make claims about products. The FDA is concerned that DSHEA will weaken its ability to protect the American public from unsafe products.)

The claims that health food companies make about their products are usually based on research performed by other parties, frequently scientists at universities not affiliated with or supported by the health food companies. Because they don't perform their own research, these companies can sell their products at a lower cost (which is good for the consumer). But because they do not support research, they do not develop substantially new or more effective therapies (which is not good for the consumer), and they generally do not subject their products to rigorous testing, which is one of the reasons that the medical community is skeptical of dietary supplements.

Finally, quality control for dietary supplements is not as rigorous as that for drugs. As a result, the many products on the market range from very good to impure or diluted. One example of this wide spectrum is the quality of fish oil capsules. A few years ago, Professor Tom Saldeen, professor and chairman at the Department of Forensic Medicine in Uppsala, Sweden, and an expert on fish, studied the antioxidant potency of fish oil capsules in health food stores. To his surprise, he found a remarkable range in antioxidant potency of various fish oil preparations, with a two-hundred-fold difference between the best and the worst products. The best products were beneficial and protected blood lipids from oxidation. By contrast, the worst products were unhealthy; he found that taking these unstable fish oils caused oxidative stress and burned up vitamin E in the blood of subjects using the inferior supplements. Another example: when the Good Housekeeping Institute analyzed six popular brands of St. John's wort supplement, they found an almost twentyfold difference in supplement potency.[3] Reporters at the *Los Angeles Times* found similar inconsistencies in the purity of St. John's wort preparations.[4]

The health food industry could use better product quality standards. And it needs to perform or support research to demonstrate the efficacy and safety of its products. To achieve these goals, the government could provide incentives. For example, companies should be allowed to make exclusive health claims for their products if they have funded or performed research that supports those claims. A "seal of approval" could be given to products that meet standards of safety, efficacy, and quality. For this to be credible, and to motivate industry, these designations of exclusivity and/or approval should be rapidly reviewed and authorized by an unbiased group composed of scientists, health professionals, consumer advocates, and industry experts. Incentives such as these will motivate industry to produce higher-quality products and to perform research that will result in new or improved products, goals that have not been fully achieved by the current legislation and regulations. Products with these designations will have a competitive advantage and can be sold at a premium. The seal of approval and/or approved health claim would be useful to consumers, and consumers would also benefit from new and improved products.

COMPARING DRUGS AND SUPPLEMENTS

Drugs	Supplements
Highly regulated	Simpler regulations
High cost	Low cost
Available only after rigorous and large clinical trials	No research required, but usually based on decades and often centuries of use by practitioners of folk medicine
High quality control	Less quality control
Well-supported claims	Claims sometimes exaggerated
Highly effective relief of symptoms	Milder action
Side effects may be harsh	Fewer side effects

AN INTERTWINED HISTORY: DRUGS AND HERBAL REMEDIES

Many herbal preparations on the market are based on hundreds, even thousands, of years of folk medicine. In fact, the creation of many modern drugs are based on some of these folk medicines. For example, digoxin, a drug commonly used for heart failure and irregular heartbeats, is based on the foxglove plant. Foxglove was widely used in medieval Europe to treat "dropsy," swelling of the body, which was often due to heart failure. Lovastatin, the basis of the class of drugs known as statins to lower cholesterol, was derived from red yeast rice, which has been used in China for centuries for "circulation" and as a flavor enhancer for foods.

Beware of Side Effects and Interactions

JUST BECAUSE herbal remedies may be slightly milder on the body, don't think that they are without side effects or can't interact with other medications. Anything you put into your body, even if it's natural, can have an adverse effect. The side effects of natural products, just as those with medications, can be due to an excessive dose or may be just the body's reaction to the product.

Each one of us is different and reacts individually to therapies, whether drugs or natural. We react based on a variety of issues: age, gender, and genetics; what we ate today; and whether or not we had a recent or chronic illness.

For example, ephedra, also known by its Chinese name mahuang, is a commonly used herbal supplement for energy and weight loss. Often taken with caffeine, ephedra increases heart rate and blood pressure. In a healthy individual, these side effects may go unnoticed. But in an individual with heart disease, these heart rate and blood pressure increases can have devastating consequences, including high blood pressure, palpitations, stroke, seizures, and even death. Over a period of two years, 140 serious adverse events with ephedra were reported to the FDA.[5] In determining which supplements may be right for you, it's important for you and your doctor to take into account your condition and current state of health.

Here are some general recommendations about the use of dietary supplements:

1. Deciding Whether You Need Supplements

· If you are healthy, you do not need nutritional supplements. You need to follow my diet and exercise program.

· If you are at risk for heart disease but feel fine, some of the supplements below may reduce your risk factors. However, they are not a replacement for a healthy diet, exercise, and appropriate medicines. None of the supplements below have been proven to prevent heart attack or stroke.

· If you have symptoms, some of the supplements below may reduce pain and make you feel better. However, these supplements are not a replacement for a healthy diet and exercise. Nor are they a replacement for medical evaluation and treatment. If you have heart or vessel disease, you need to be under the care of a physician.

2. How to Use Supplements Effectively

· Get your physician involved. It's very important that your doctor or health professional know about your use of supplements. Do not take any supplement that you haven't first discussed with your physician.

   Doctors, nurse practitioners, and other health professionals are becoming increasingly interested in, and educated about, the use of supplements. Your doctor can guide you in determining if you need a supplement and can help you choose the ones that are right for you. Your doctor can also help you evaluate the usefulness of a particular supplement or whether it has an adverse effect. *By all means, let your doctor know what supplements you are taking. If your doctor is not interested in this information, then you may need a new doctor.*[6]

· Find the best product. Not all supplements are of the same quality. Unfortunately, there is no widely accepted evaluation process for guaranteeing the quality of supplements, so buyer beware! In general, products manufactured and distributed by the largest health food companies and pharmaceutical companies are probably better choices if no other information is available. These companies have a brand to protect and take extra care to avoid ruining their reputations. One good source of information on the quality of supplements is www.consumerlab.com.

· Use one supplement at a time. If you are trying out supplements, by all means, use one at a time. Don't end up taking handfuls of supplements hoping that you are going to make yourself healthy. Put each of the supplements through a rigorous test. By adopting a systematic method for taking supplements, you will ensure that you are not wasting your time or money on ineffective supplements.

I generally recommend that patients take one supplement regularly for a month. If you are feeling better, and/or if symptoms improve during that month, and/or if a specific biomarker has improved (i.e., cholesterol), continue to take the supplement. If you do not feel better or the symptoms have not improved, then you may need to increase the dose. If the supplement doesn't seem to be working at the highest dose or you have developed some new symptoms (which could be a side effect), then stop the supplement and try something else. If the supplement doesn't work for you, or if you have any of the side effects described, don't waste any more of your money on it. (See the self-evaluation method on p. 232.)

Following is a list of supplements that can be tried for various heart and vessel problems.

SUPPLEMENTS FOR SYMPTOMS

For angina:
L-arginine
L-carnitine
Ginkgo biloba

For difficulty walking because of poor circulation:
L-arginine
L-carnitine
Ginkgo biloba

For shortness of breath and poor exercise tolerance due to a weak heart:
Coenzyme Q10
L-arginine

For painful veins or leg swelling:
Grape seed extract
Horse chestnut seed extract

For circulatory instability (hot flashes):
Phytoestrogens (daidzein and genistein)

SUPPLEMENTS FOR TREATING RISK FACTORS

For reducing trigylceride levels:
Fish oil supplementation

For controlling blood sugar:
Chromium picolinate (possibly effective)

For reducing cholesterol:
Garlic
Policosanol (possibly effective)
Vitamin B_3 (niacin)
Sterol- or stanol-containing margarine substitutes

For reducing homocysteine levels:
Vitamins B_6, B_{12}, and folate

For lowering blood pressure:
Potassium salt substitutes

Supplements

L-ARGININE

Description: Amino acid.

Use: For people with symptoms of heart or vessel disease, including

- chest pain due to coronary artery blockages
- leg cramping due to narrowing in the leg arteries
- shortness of breath, difficulty walking, or fatigue due to a weak heart
- impotence

From our research, and that of other labs around the world, we have found that many people benefit from supplemental L-arginine.

In people with heart and vessel disease, L-arginine restores production of NO and improves blood flow—and, in so doing, relieves symptoms of heart and vessel disease. It can increase exercise tolerance and improve sexual performance in men who have vasculogenic impotence (impotence due to poor penile blood flow, the most common cause of erectile dysfunction).

Dose: 3 to 9 grams daily in equally divided doses.

Why do you need so much L-arginine? Your intestine and liver are chock-full of an enzyme, arginase, that breaks down L-arginine. After passing through the intestine and liver, only about 40 to 50 percent of the L-arginine you ingest actually reaches the vessels in the rest of your body. Another reason high doses are needed is that L-arginine gets diverted to other pathways besides the NO synthase pathway. L-arginine is used to make a number of substances in the body, including the neurotransmitter agmatine. Finally, you need to have adequate blood levels of L-arginine to overcome the elevation of ADMA. (People with vascular disease have high levels of ADMA, which interferes with production of NO; but these high levels can be reduced with supplemental L-arginine.)

Side effects: Stomach upset, diarrhea, headache, recurrence of cold sores or shingles. Side effects are rare. Adverse interactions with other drugs have not been reported, but have not been thoroughly studied. L-arginine should not be used with Viagra since blood pressure might drop too low. However, there have been no reports of this adverse event.

Who should not use: L-arginine is not recommended for patients with cancer or a history of cancer. If is not yet clear from studies whether L-arginine makes existing tumors grow faster or whether it provides an antitumor benefit. L-arginine does not cause cancer.

L-arginine is not recommended for patients with a serious infection (such as in someone who is being hospitalized) or patients with inflammation (such as systemic lupus erythematosus or rheumatoid arthritis). In serious infections, there can be an overproduction of nitric oxide, causing low blood pressure. In severe inflammatory conditions, a local overproduction of nitric oxide may contribute to the inflammation.

L-CARNITINE

Description: Modified amino acid.

Use: For people with symptoms of heart or vessel disease:

- chest pain with exertion
- shortness of breath
- aching of the legs while walking

L-carnitine is a modified amino acid used by the body to create energy from fat. L-carnitine carries fatty acids into the mitochondria (the cell furnace that burns fuel to create energy). Without healthy amounts of L-carnitine, the body can't produce enough energy.

The body needs vitamin B_6, vitamin C, niacin, and iron to make L-carnitine. Normally, the body makes enough L-carnitine. But in certain conditions, levels of this modified amino acid are low in, for example, areas of the heart or leg muscle where there is not enough blood flow. The lack of L-carnitine leads to an accumulation of fatty acid and results in insufficient energy. This situation can be reversed with L-carnitine supplementation.

Dose: 1.5 to 6 grams daily.

Side effects: Stomach upset, nausea, diarrhea. Side effects are rare.

COENZYME Q10

Description: Cofactor for energy generation. Antioxidant.

Use: Congestive heart failure or weak heart.

Coenzyme Q10 (CoQ10) is an antioxidant made by the body that helps vitamins C and E to detoxify superoxide anion. CoQ10 also reduces the oxidation of cholesterol in the blood vessel wall.

CoQ10 is widely used in Europe and Japan. The best data to support its use come from clinical trials in patients with heart failure. In these individuals, CoQ10 improves shortness of breath and reduces hospitalizations. (Several medications reduce levels of CoQ10, notably the statins or cholesterol-lowering medications. Some nutritionists add CoQ10 to the regimen of patients taking statins.)

However, there is no evidence that CoQ10 prevents heart attack or stroke.

Dose: 30 to 150 milligrams daily.

Side effects: Occasionally causes stomach upset.

CHROMIUM PICOLINATE

Description: Mineral.

Use: Possibly helpful in restoring healthy levels of blood sugar and insulin. Several studies have shown that in people with insulin resistance syndrome, or Type 2 diabetes mellitus, chromium supplementation may improve blood sugar control and reduce the need for diabetes medication. It may slightly reduce LDL cholesterol and triglycerides and increase HDL cholesterol.

Trace amounts of chromium are necessary for proper control of blood sugar. It is best to obtain chromium through a balanced diet; potatoes, whole wheat bread, green peppers, and brewer's yeast are all good sources of chromium. (Chromium is generally marketed as chromium picolinate.)

Dose: 50 to 200 micrograms daily.

Side effects: Rare reports of heavy metal toxicity at higher doses. At higher doses, there have been a few reports of serious side effects, including adverse effects on the blood, kidneys, and liver.

Who should not use: Chromium picolinate should not be used by individuals who have severe emotional disorders, since picolinate may have an adverse effect on brain function in these individuals.

FISH OIL SUPPLEMENTATION
(OMEGA-3 FATTY ACIDS DHA AND EPA)

Description: Omega-3 fatty acids.

Use: To reduce high triglyceride levels.

Most people could use more fish in their diet (particularly fatty fish such as mackerel, herring, or salmon). Supplementation with omega-3 from fish oil or algae can also help. Omega-3 fatty acids can improve endothelial health; they also reduce triglycerides, keep blood from clotting too quickly, and have anti-inflammatory properties.

When selecting a fish oil supplement, it's important to choose carefully. Many fish oil supplements in health food stores are not worth buying. Because fish oils are very unsaturated, they tend to become oxidized or rancid very easily. Oxidized fish oil is not good for you; it can generate free radicals and consume your body's stores of vitamin E. If you have diabetes, rancid fish oil could increase your blood sugar.

Determine if your fish oil supplement is oxidized by biting through the capsule and tasting it. Oxidized fish oil has an unpleasant or fishy odor and taste. By contrast, high-quality fish oil has no taste or odor.

During the processing of fish oils, the environmental contaminants that are concentrated in fish are removed. Unfortunately, because of water pollution, unprocessed fish oil contains traces of heavy metals (cadmium, copper, iron, magnesium, and lead), which can be toxic. Fish oil may also contain traces of pesticides, such as DDT and PCB. Commercial processing of fish oil removes these contaminants, but also removes the natural antioxidants that keep fish oil from becoming rancid. Most commercial suppliers add antioxidants back to the fish oil (most commonly, vitamin E), but the presence of vitamin E alone does not ensure stability. Stability testing reveals great differences between fish oil preparations.

To avoid the problems with commercial processing of fish oils, some manufacturers are now obtaining EPA and DHA from algae. Algae are single-cell organisms found in the water that are eaten by fish. In fact, the EPA and DHA in fish come from their diet of algae. Some manufacturers are now growing algae and isolating the omega-3s from these microscopic organisms. The advantage of this approach is that the algae are grown free of contamination by heavy metals and pesticides.

Dose: At Stanford, we recommend 1 to 2 grams of fish oil daily for people with high triglycerides. Occasionally, we use a combination of fish oil and garlic supplementation, which has been shown to be more helpful in lowering cholesterol levels than either one alone.

Sometimes patients will also need niacin or the drug gemfibrozil to further reduce triglycerides.

Side effects: Stomach upset, gas.

Who should not use: Because omega-3s have a slight tendency to reduce blood clot formation, people with bleeding tendencies (such as hemophiliacs) should not use these supplements. Individuals who are already taking aspirin or blood thinners should proceed with caution and be attentive to any sign that their blood is too thin (bleeding gums, easy bruising). If you develop bleeding gums or experience easy bruising, then stop using this supplement until you speak to your doctor.

GARLIC (ALLICIN)

Description: Herb or herbal extract.

Use: Reducing cholesterol.

One way to supplement your diet with garlic is to cook with one clove daily. Garlic in pill form is a safe alternative. Garlic is healthy for the heart and vessels for several reasons. It is known to reduce cholesterol; it lowers blood pressure and produces a mild antiplatelet activity, mainly because it increases the activity of NO synthase. Garlic may help "clear the arteries," as proposed by Dioscorides in the first century A.D.

In addition, garlic has antibacterial properties. During World War II, it was known as "Russian penicillin" after the Soviet government turned to garlic after exhausting its supply of antibiotics. Garlic may also have anticancer benefits; in one large study of about 42,000 women, those who consumed more garlic in their diet were 30 percent less likely to develop colon cancer.

Garlic contains a number of factors that may be healthful, but much of its benefit can be attributed to a protein called allicin that gives garlic its smell and sharp taste. Until the clove is crushed, activating a protein called alliinase, allicin exists mainly as an odorless compound called alliin.

Allicin is not very stable; it disintegrates after three hours at room temperature, or with 20 minutes of cooking. For this reason, there is very little allicin in garlic powder. (Because allicin is unstable, pill manufacturers make the pill so that when it is swallowed, it mixes with moisture in the stomach and the allicin is released.)

In the health food store, there are many garlic products, including dried, aged, or deodorized garlic preparations and garlic oil. They contain varying amounts of allicin. Garlic oil does not contain any allicin and has very little lipid-lowering benefit. The differences in these products may account for the varying effectiveness observed in clinical trials.

Dose: Alliin, 10 milligrams daily (5 milligrams allicin daily). If you want to use a garlic product, try a deodorized powder; the label should indicate the amount of alliin per tablet.

Side effects: Body odor, upset stomach, flushing.

GINKGO BILOBA

Description: Herbal extract.

Use: For leg pain due to poor circulation or peripheral arterial disease (PAD).

Extracts of the leaves of ginkgo biloba trees have been used therapeutically for centuries in Chinese traditional medicine. Several clinical trials have indicated that extracts of ginkgo can improve mental functioning in people with Alzheimer's disease. EGb 761 is a highly standardized extract of ginkgo biloba leaves commonly used by physicians in Europe for treatment of PAD.

A variety of commercially produced ginkgo extracts (often of uncertain standardization) is increasing in the United States. However, the standardized extract EGb 761 is now available in the U.S. in several commercial products.

Dose: 160 to 320 milligrams daily.

Side effects: Generally, patients don't have very much problem with ginkgo biloba. There have been a few cases of bleeding associated with the use of ginkgo in people taking medications that affect blood clotting (aspirin or Coumadin). If you are taking one of these, use ginkgo with caution. If you develop more noticeable bruising or have any excessive bleeding, then this supplement should be discontinued until you speak to your doctor.

GRAPE SEED EXTRACT

Description: Herbal extract.

Use: Leg swelling due to vein or lymph disease.

Grape seed extract is widely used in France (where the majority of clinical trials have been performed) to reduce swelling that accompanies vein or lymph disease (see discussion of horse chestnut seed extract below). Grape seed extract contains oligomeric proanthocyanidins (OPCs), which are the main active ingredients. These are capable of reducing the leakage of fluid out of vessels. As antioxidants, OPCs can function in a similar manner to vitamin C and can prevent the breakdown of collagen. (Also found in pine bark, OPCs were introduced to French explorers by Native Americans who used tea made from pine bark to prevent scurvy.)

OPCs are also found in hawthorn, onions, legumes, berries, and parsley. The best way to obtain OPCs, and related flavonoids, is by increasing the fruit and vegetables in your diet. Black tea, wine, and grape juice are also excellent sources of flavonoids.

Dose: 150 to 300 milligrams daily of the active ingredient OPC.

Side effects: Nontoxic in this dose range.

HORSE CHESTNUT SEED EXTRACT

Description: Herbal extract.

Use: Reduce leg pain and swelling due to vein or lymph disease.

At the Vascular Medicine Clinic at Stanford, we regularly recommend horse chestnut seed extract to people with venous insufficiency or lymphedema, swelling of the limb due to blockages in the lymphatic vessels draining that limb. The lymphatics are small vessels that return fluid in the tissues back to circulation. Venous insufficiency is a condition caused by clots in the veins or leaking of the valves of the veins. The condition, which is unrelated to hardening of the arteries, occurs when the veins aren't working properly; leg pain or varicose veins may develop. However, sometimes people develop this condition when a leg vein is removed during surgery to be used as a bypass of a blocked artery. Horse chestnut seed extract works by reducing inflammation and the leakage of fluid out of the veins. It has been used safely in Europe for years.

Dose: 50 to 100 milligrams twice daily of the active ingredient escin.

Side effects: Minimal, but could include nausea and kidney and liver problems.

POLICOSANOL

Description: A waxy substance made usually from sugarcane.

Use: Possibly helpful in reducing cholesterol.

This is an herbal supplement that has been shown to be somewhat effective in reducing cholesterol. A waxy substance, it is generally manufactured from sugarcane and is also found in wheat germ oil and alfalfa, as is the related substance octacosanol. Randomized clinical trials involving over 1,500 people have shown that in doses of 5 to 10 milligrams twice daily, policosanol reduces LDL cholesterol by over 20 percent. However, most of these studies have originated from one lab in Cuba, and confirmatory studies are needed.

Dose: 5 to 10 milligrams once or twice daily.

Side effects: It may have a mild antiplatelet effect, so should be used cautiously with aspirin, Coumadin, or other drugs or supplements that can thin the blood.

SOY SUPPLEMENTS

Description: Phytoestrogens.

Use: To improve vascular relaxation (and reduce hot flashes).

The phytochemicals in soy, otherwise known as phytoestrogens, have been shown to improve heart and blood vessel health. Soy phytoestrogens, also called isoflavones, are antioxidants and anti-inflammatories. The isoflavones in particular that seem to be of greatest benefit are genistein and daidzein. The best way to get these into your diet is to eat soy products. However, if you don't like soy, soy supplements are an alternative.

Soy supplements can be taken to reduce the symptoms of menopause. And they can be taken to improve vessel relaxation. In a recent study conducted at Stanford, we examined the effect of a soy supplement on the health of the blood vessels of postmenopausal women with high cholesterol. Half of the women in our study were given 50 milligrams of soy isoflavones (genistein, daidzein, and glycitein) once daily. After several weeks we examined their blood vessels—and found a marked improvement in the ability of the blood vessels to relax as compared to the control group who received placebo.

Soy isoflavones may protect LDL cholesterol from oxidation. The isoflavones may destroy free radicals and superoxide anion. The enzymes we need to control free oxygen radicals are also favorably affected by isoflavones.

Dose: 25 to 75 milligrams of phytoestrogen (daidzein/genistein/glycitein mixture) daily or 25 to 75 grams of soy protein (about 1 to 3 ounces of soy protein).

Side effects: None known.

Who should not use: Women who have had breast cancer should consult with their physician before using soy supplements.

VITAMIN B₃ (NIACIN)

Description: Vitamin.

Use: To lower bad cholesterol and increase good cholesterol.

Vitamin B_3 is used by the body to create energy or fat from carbohydrates. It is also needed to metabolize alcohol. The best food sources of vitamin B_3 are peanuts, brewer's yeast, fish, and meat, and (to a lesser extent) whole grains.

Vitamin B_3 comes in two forms—niacin (also called nicotinic acid) and niacinamide (also called nicotinamide). Niacin (but not niacinamide) in high doses can lower cholesterol. (Because it has few side effects, inositol hexaniacinate is sometimes prescribed by European doctors for those who need high doses of niacin.)

Dose: 50 to 2000 milligrams daily. High doses (over 100 milligrams daily) of niacin or inositol hexaniacinate should be taken only under the direct supervision of a doctor.

Niacin in amounts as low as 50 to 100 milligrams may cause flushing, headache, and stomachache. Doctors sometimes prescribe very high amounts of niacin (1 to 3 grams per day) to reduce LDL choles-

THE PROS AND CONS OF PRESCRIBING NIACIN

How to decide between taking a statin or niacin? I usually make a recommendation based on each individual patient. Statins have few side effects, and so are easy to prescribe. Many physicians don't like to prescribe niacin because of its minor but annoying side effects (a sensation of warmth and redness of the skin called flushing and/or stomach upset). But niacin is a vitamin, and many patients may prefer a natural substance. Niacin, which can also increase HDL cholesterol to a greater extent than most statin drugs, is less expensive than statins.

To reduce the stomach upset and flushing that occur with niacin, start out with a low dose (50 to 100 milligrams three times daily) after meals. If you still have flushing, take a baby aspirin (81 milligrams) before each meal. After a week, double the dose of niacin to 100 to 200 milligrams three times daily. After six to eight weeks you need a blood test to check cholesterol levels, triglycerides, and liver enzymes (you need the latter test because all cholesterol-lowering agents, even natural ones, have the potential to affect your liver).

If healthy cholesterol and triglyceride levels are not obtained with this dose, it can be doubled to 200 to 400 milligrams three times daily under a doctor's guidance. The dose can be increased to up to 3 grams per day, although most people have to stop at about 2 grams per day because of flushing and stomach upset. Alternatively, your doctor can prescribe a sustained-release form of niacin that may be more expensive but only has to be taken once a day and typically causes less flushing and stomach upset.

terol and to increase HDL cholesterol. Generally these high doses of niacin are safe, but are often accompanied by flushing and stomach upset. These large amounts can cause liver damage, make diabetes worse, cause irritation of the stomach, and increase blood levels of uric acid (which can cause gout). These side effects can be detected by your doctor at an early stage and can be reversed by reducing the amount of niacin that you are taking or stopping it altogether.

Side effects: Flushing, stomach upset, liver problems.

VITAMINS B$_6$, B$_{12}$, AND FOLATE

Description: B-complex vitamins.

Use: To reduce homocysteine levels.

The B vitamins—B$_6$, B$_{12}$, and folate (folic acid)—work in our body as cofactors helping the function of certain enzymes. They play an important role in cardiovascular health. The Nurses' Health Study demonstrated that women who consume more B vitamins (either from food or vitamins) had half the risk of heart disease as those who ingested less B vitamins. And B vitamins are needed so that the body can rid itself of homocysteine, which is toxic at high levels and a risk factor for cardiovascular disease.

Homocysteine levels are often too high in people who have kidney or liver impairment, in people who have some genetic disorders, and in those who are deficient in B vitamins.

How, one might ask, can there be a nutritional deficiency in the citizens of a country that is the most well fed in the world? The answer is simple. Americans are eating the wrong foods. Homocysteine is derived from methionine, an amino acid that is found in higher amounts in animal protein. If you eat a diet high in animal protein and low in fruits and vegetables, then your homocysteine level goes up. If you can't increase your B vitamins through nutrition (by eating enriched grains; see nutrient lists at end of Chapter 4), you may need supplementation.

Dose: 10 to 25 milligrams daily B$_6$; 400 micrograms to 1 milligram daily of folate.

Most people who eat a healthy diet do not need B$_{12}$ vitamins. However, vegetarians and the elderly (who have less ability to absorb the vitamin from the foods they eat) may benefit from 100 to 200 micrograms daily. If you are anemic (low blood count, have numbness or tingling in your hands or feet, or have sores at the corner of the mouth), you may have B_{12} deficiency.

Side effects: Very safe when taken together. At very high doses (200 milligrams or more daily) B_6 can damage nerves, leading to numbness in the hands and feet and difficulty walking. Stop B_6 if any of these symptoms develop.

VITAMINS C AND E

Description: Antioxidant vitamins.

Use: Prevention of heart attack and stroke (but not well-supported by clinical trials).

It may surprise you that I do not actively recommend vitamin E or vitamin C. I used to recommend high doses (400 international units or IU of vitamin E and 500 milligrams of vitamin C). I no longer recommend these high doses, for three reasons. First, there is a lot of data from recent large and well-controlled clinical trials such as the Heart Outcomes Prevention Evaluation (HOPE) study and the MRC/BHF Heart Protection Study (funded by the UK's Medical Research Council, MRC), and British Heart Foundation (BHF) that do not support the use of high-dose antioxidant vitamins to prevent heart disease.

Second, there are some recent reports of increased bleeding in patients taking high doses of antioxidant vitamins with blood-thinning medications. Since most patients with heart disease need to be on antiplatelet medicine, they may be at higher risk for bleeding if they use high-dose antioxidant vitamins. Furthermore, there is a very recent study that shows that antioxidant vitamins at high doses (beta-carotene at 12.5 milligrams twice a day, vitamin C at 500 milligrams twice a day, vitamin E at 400 IU twice a day, and selenium at 50 micrograms twice a day) can blunt the beneficial effects of statins to increase HDL cholesterol.[7] Finally, in light of negative studies with high doses of a single antioxidant vitamin, it seems best to obtain a variety of antioxidants through diet, rather than large amounts of one antioxidant vitamin. Generous and frequent servings of fruits and vegetables, as many as seven to nine daily, can give a wide and balanced variety of natural antioxidants, some of which are even more potent than vitamins E and C.

Dose: If you want to supplement with vitamins E and C, I would recommend that you take a lower dose than is generally used—no more than 100 IU of vitamin E and 100 milligrams of vitamin C daily. My recommendations are in keeping with the current Recommended Daily Allowances established by the government (15 micrograms for vitamin E and 90 milligrams for vitamin C). You will obtain this amount of antioxidant protection by adhering to the diet I have outlined.

Both vitamin C and vitamin E have been shown to reduce the breakdown of nitric oxide and to enhance its vessel-relaxing properties. In people with diabetes, vitamin C improves endothelium-dependent relaxation of blood vessels. In people with high levels of cholesterol, and in people with coronary artery disease, vitamin E has been shown to improve vessel relaxation. The positive benefit of vitamins E and C on vessel relaxation and blood flow are due to their protection of NO. Furthermore, populations who consume high amounts of vitamins E and C have less coronary artery disease (but this may also be due to the fact that these same individuals consume more plant antioxidants in their diet and have a generally healthy lifestyle). In addition, people taking vitamins C and E have platelets that are less sticky and cholesterol that is less easily oxidized.

Over the years, however, there has been some controversy about how much vitamin C is healthy and how much is too much. Most notable in the controversy was the scientist Linus Pauling (a maverick who won a Nobel Peace Prize in 1962 for an internationally successful campaign to end nuclear bomb testing and a Nobel Prize in Chemistry in 1954 for his research on the nature of the chemical bond).

In the 1970s and 1980s, Pauling turned his attention to a different battle: nutritional medicine. He became an advocate for megadoses of vitamin C as a way of boosting the immune system and curing diseases such as cancer and atherosclerosis. At that time, Pauling recommended that people take up to 18 grams (18,000 milligrams), which was 200 times the amount currently suggested by the RDA.

Today, even the Linus Pauling Institute in Palo Alto has changed its recommendation, acknowledging that 18 grams is simply too much vitamin C for the body to handle. Vitamin C does play an important role in health (similar to what Pauling believed, but in lesser amounts). Vitamin C is important to collagen formation, which strengthens bones, muscles, and blood vessels. It is also used by the body for regular tissue repair and growth during wound healing.

However, too much vitamin C doesn't do the body any good. Excessive amounts are excreted when the body has too much, and renal stones are a concern with chronic high-dose vitamin C. There is no evidence that high-dose vitamin C reduces hardening of the arteries.

Megadoses of vitamin E became popular for people with heart disease after the publication of the Cambridge Heart Antioxidant Study (CHAOS) a few years ago. About 2,000 people with atherosclerosis were studied. Participants who took 400 to 800 IU of vitamin E daily decreased their risk of heart attack and death from heart disease. Other studies have shown that vitamin E intake through diet is just as effective. One study found that postmenopausal women with high amounts of natural vitamin E in their diet had less risk of heart disease than those on vitamin E supplements. Smaller doses of vitamin E may be more effective. In a study of over 30,000 physicians, those who consumed 200 IU of vitamin E daily had about a 40 percent reduction in heart attack. There didn't seem to be any greater benefit of higher vitamin E consumption.

More recently, the Heart Outcomes Prevention Evaluation (HOPE) study followed 10,000 patients for four and a half years. The patients, who were at high risk for heart attack or stroke, received 265 milligrams (400 IU) of vitamin E daily. As it turned out, these patients did not have fewer heart attacks and strokes compared to those who did not take the supplement, leaving researchers to question the benefit of vitamin E supplements. It is possible, however, that this trial failed to show a benefit of antioxidant therapy because only vitamin E was used. A combination of antioxidant substances is likely to be more effective than high doses of vitamins E or C alone.

To summarize, the best way to increase your daily dose of antioxidants is with seven to nine daily servings of fruits and vegetables. If you want to take supplements of vitamins E and C, use the lower doses that I have recommended above, since some data show that low doses may be helpful, whereas higher doses may be counterproductive.

Side effects: None at this dose range.

Medical and Functional Foods

MEDICAL FOODS are a type of nutritional intervention in a class all their own. Regulated by the FDA, these foods were established as such by the Orphan Drug Act of 1988. Nutritionally designed for a specific disease, they can be used as a nutritional addition to medical therapy, and only under the supervision of a health professional.

There are several medical foods for heart and vessel disease that may be useful in your program of heart and vessel health. I created one of these, the HeartBar.

Functional foods are considered to be foods by the FDA, but have been developed for the purpose of meeting a specific health need.

BENECOL, TAKE CONTROL

Description: Plant-based products containing sterols.

Use: Lowers cholesterol.

These functional foods can be spread on toast or bagels—just as you would spread butter or margarine. Designed to reduce cholesterol levels, these medical foods are very popular in Finland. These margarines contain plant sterols that taste and look very similar to cholesterol but can't be absorbed as well. The plant sterols in these products also associate with cholesterol in your intestine and help your body excrete cholesterol.

Take Control (Lipton) uses an extract of the soy plant, sitosterol. An extract of pine needles, sitostanol is available in a similar product called Benecol (McNeil). I have used Benecol and find that it tastes quite good, similar to margarine. Spreading 1 to 2 tablespoons of Benecol on bread each day, as a substitute for margarine, can reduce LDL cholesterol levels by up to 10 percent and can enhance the effects of statins.

Dose: 1 to 3 tablespoons daily.

Side effects: Not many. Occasionally some gastric upset.

CARDIA SALT

Description: Salt replacement.

Use: Lowers blood pressure.

Cardia Salt contains 50 percent less sodium per serving than regular table salt. The sodium is replaced by potassium, magnesium, and lysine. Potassium and magnesium help to maintain a normal heartbeat and reduce blood pressure. There is a lot of data from clinical trials that increasing potassium in the diet can reduce blood pressure. There is also good evidence to suggest that potassium and magnesium can stabilize the heart rhythm. Two clinical trials using Cardia Salt show that it helps in the dietary management of high blood pressure.

Dose: Use instead of salt to flavor food.

Side effects: Minimal. Use under medical supervision if you are taking medicines that reduce potassium excretion (Aldactone, ACE inhibitors, angiotensin II antagonists).

HEARTBAR

Description: L-arginine-enriched medical food.

Use: For symptoms of heart and vessel disease.

I found L-arginine to be effective in treating heart and vessel problems so I founded Cooke Pharma (www.cookepharma.com), a company that develops cardiovascular medical foods. We embarked on a mission to create a nutritional therapy that would take advantage of the recent research into nutrients and endothelial health.

We designed the HeartBar, one of the first medical foods specifically designed for cardiovascular health, so that patients would have an easy way of getting many of the nutrients for their heart and vessels in a good-tasting health bar. In clinical trials, the bar has been shown to improve endothelial health, increase blood flow, and improve exercise tolerance in heart patients.

Besides L-arginine, the HeartBar contains the antioxidant vitamins C and E, which preserve nitric oxide; vitamins B_6, B_{12}, and folate, which reduce blood homocysteine levels; and soy protein, which

HOW THE HEARTBAR HAS HELPED
SOME OF MY PATIENTS

Mr. Larry Moitozo is a vigorous and energetic 78-year-old from Los Gatos, California, who looks 15 years younger. Now retired, Larry had been an environmental biologist and professor at UC Santa Cruz and San Jose State. His favorite course had been alpine biology, the study of plants and animals in the mountains. Each year, he had taken students hiking for a month through Yosemite and King's Canyon. Even in retirement, Larry spent his vacations trekking all over the world and enjoying the outdoors with his son.

In the last few years, though, Larry began to experience some cramping in his legs after walking up a hill. The discomfort would subside if he stood still for a moment, and then he could go on. But about two years ago, the cramping began to really bother him. His legs would tighten up after walking a half mile, and often he could go that far only if he walked slowly. The great outdoors was getting farther away for Larry.

Larry came to my Vascular Medicine Clinic at Stanford in the spring of 1999. I recognized his symptoms as peripheral arterial disease (PAD), a form of atherosclerosis that affects the arteries of the leg. I started him on the available drug therapy for PAD. He returned to me six weeks later with little improvement. At that point, I stopped the drug therapy and introduced him to my program for endothelial health and the L-arginine-enriched bar. Larry began taking two bars daily. It wasn't long before he noticed an improvement in his ability to walk. At the time of this writing, Larry is able to walk faster, without pain, and considers himself unlimited. He is even able to jog a quarter of a mile before he needs to slow down. He's back to the hills, and enjoying the outdoors again with his son.

My program for endothelial health has also helped patients with angina and chest pain due to coronary heart disease. Mr. Mohsen Mikhail is a busy chief executive officer and founder of an educational company. His work involves overseeing the administration of four vocational schools. Although he has been very successful, his success has come at a cost. Mr. Mikhail's job is stressful, and his high blood pressure, high cholesterol, and diabetes have, over the years, taken a toll on his heart. In 1979 he had a triple bypass and stopped smoking. After that, he had two heart attacks and multiple angioplasties.

When he first came to my clinic in 1995 suffering from chest pain, I increased his medical therapy and got his blood pressure, diabetes, and high cholesterol under control. However, despite the best medical therapy, he showed up in my clinic again in 1998 with more chest pain. Coronary angiography revealed that his by-pass grafts had narrowed and that his heart arteries had shrunk to such a degree that another bypass operation would be difficult. He was already on maximal medical therapy, taking nitroglycerin pills about three to six times daily for breakthrough chest pain. I told Mr. Mikhail about my program for endothelial health and the diet and exercise changes that he would need to improve his vascular health. I also asked him to try the L-arginine-enriched bar.

At his next visit to me a couple of weeks later, Mr. Mikhail was radiant. The angina had improved markedly. He rarely needed to use nitroglycerin. He was even able to get back to his old work schedule and is now enjoying life with less pain.

contains antioxidants as well as phytoestrogens (which also enhance vessel relaxation). The bar, which also has fiber and a small amount of niacin, comes in several flavors, including peanut butter, cran-berry, and vanilla, and is an excellent replacement for unhealthy snacks. It is also available as a drink mix.

Dose: One to two bars daily.

Side effects: Gastrointestinal upset, headache.

Supplements That Could Be Useful

THERE ARE a few supplements that I do not currently recommend. This is mainly because they don't have enough scientific support or enough of a track record in this country. They deserve more study because of their potential benefit to the heart and vessels.

Red yeast rice has been used in China for centuries as a flavor en-hancer, food preservative, and medicine. Red yeast is grown on rice and contains a number of substances that reduce cholesterol levels in the blood. The drug lovastatin (Mevacor) acts in a similar way as the ingredients in red yeast rice. Red yeast rice has been clinically proven to reduce cholesterol in human trials. A dose of red yeast rice of 2.4 grams daily has been shown to reduce cholesterol about 15 to 20 percent. In the United States, red yeast rice is no longer available. The FDA has placed restrictions on it because it has been ruled to be a drug. There is another problem with red yeast rice, that of purity (which of course is a generic problem for the entire health food industry). A UCLA study showed that only one of nine red yeast rice supplements in health food stores contained all the monacolins that lower cholesterol. Seven of nine brands contained a small amount of a toxic by-product of the fermentation process. Red yeast rice should not be combined with erythromycin, other statin drugs, the class of drugs called fibrates, or high-dose niacin. Serious side effects (such as myositis, which is muscle inflammation, or liver problems) are more likely when combined with these medications.

Guggulsterone (guggul) is an ancient Indian herbal medicine, a gum derived from the myrrh tree. It has been approved for use in India to reduce cholesterol, and in a standardized dose of 100 milligrams, guggulsterone reduces cholesterol by about 10 percent. There are not as many randomized clinical trials documenting its effectiveness and safety in reducing cholesterol as there are for the other supplements mentioned in this book.

Lipoic acid is an endogenous antioxidant in the body. Normally, the body makes enough without the need for supplementation. However, in some conditions, such as diabetes, tissue lipoic acid levels are reduced. In Europe, this supplement has been used in doses of 300 to 600 milligrams daily, in the treatment of diabetic neuropathy (pain due to a nerve disorder in diabetics).

Selenium, a trace mineral, plays an important role in our antioxidant system. Nevertheless, I do not prescribe it because there is no evidence to indicate that supplemental selenium can prevent heart attack or stroke, nor is there evidence to indicate that it can improve symptoms of heart disease (except in people who live in certain parts of the world where there is not much selenium in the soil).

Selenium, which is essential for normal functioning of the immune system and thyroid gland, is also necessary for the activity of an antioxidant enzyme called glutathione peroxidase. Plants are the major source of selenium; nuts (particularly Brazil nuts) are the best source, followed by yeast, whole grains, and seafood.

The amount of selenium in soil determines how much selenium is in plants. Soils in some parts of China and Russia have very low amounts, and selenium deficiency is common in these areas. People with selenium deficiency often have weak and enlarged hearts.

The soil in the United States has enough selenium, and it is particularly abundant in the high plains of northern Nebraska and the Dakotas. The Recommended Dietary Allowance (RDA) of selenium is 55 micrograms daily (70 micrograms daily for pregnant or lactating women), and most Americans get this amount in their diet.

Although there is no compelling evidence that more selenium will prevent heart disease, there is data from a well-controlled clinical trial that selenium (200 micrograms daily) can protect against cancer. (See Information for Your Doctor, p. 289.) Too much selenium (more than 400 micrograms daily) can cause selenosis; symptoms include stomach upset, hair loss, white blotchy nails, and mild nerve damage.

D-ribose is a naturally occurring sugar, and is an integral portion of the ATP molecule, which is the body's fuel. When the heart muscle does not get enough oxygen, ATP can become depleted. Animal studies have shown that supplemental ribose can increase the heart's production of ATP after the heart has been deprived of blood flow for short periods of time. A small clinical study has shown that high doses of ribose can improve the heart's tolerance of exercise (as shown by EKG recordings). More studies need to be done to show that this treatment is effective and safe, before I begin to recommend it.

Hawthorn is approved for use in Europe for mild heart failure. In the Middle Ages, hawthorn or foxglove extracts were used to treat "dropsy," which was in most cases accumulation of fluid due to heart failure. Over time, foxglove preparations became standard therapy for heart failure; digoxin, a medication routinely used today for heart failure, is a derivative.

By contrast, hawthorn did not achieve this level of respectability in modern medicine, despite the fact that it appears to be as effective as, and is less toxic than, digoxin. This historical paradox is probably explained by the fact that the active principle of foxglove was easily isolated and could be developed into a drug. By contrast, there are a number of components in hawthorn that contribute to its beneficial effect. It has some antioxidant properties and causes a mild relaxation of the heart arteries, possibly by preserving nitric oxide. Typically, a preparation of dried flowers is used, sometimes together with the fruits and leaves as well. U.S. investigators are now examining the utility of hawthorn for cardiovascular disease.

Supplements to Avoid if You Have Heart or Vessel Disease

Vitamin A (beta-carotene), an antioxidant vitamin, is not recommended by me as a supplement for people with, or at risk for, heart disease. In smokers, vitamin A can actually increase lung cancer risk.

Because beta-carotene has antioxidant effects, it was thought that supplements might reduce heart and vessel disease. But large, randomized clinical trials showed otherwise. The results of these studies (and the large studies with vitamin E that have shown no benefit on heart disease) indicate that large doses of antioxidant vitamins are not useful, and in fact may be harmful.

On the other hand, studies show that people live longer and have fewer heart attacks and stroke when their *diet* includes a large amount and variety of natural antioxidants. Therefore, the best source of antioxidant vitamins is in fruits and vegetables. Carrots, tomatoes, and other red and orange vegetables contain potent antioxidant carotenoids (similar to vitamin A). Liver, dairy products, and cod-liver oil also provide vitamin A.

Ephedra is possibly the worst supplement you could take if you have heart or vessel disease. Used medically by the Chinese for over 5,000 years, it is an herbal preparation that comes from a shrublike plant found in desert regions throughout the world (in particular northern China and Inner Mongolia).

Ephedra contains some potent ingredients, including ephedrine and pseudoephedrine. (You probably recognize these chemicals; small amounts of ephedrine and pseudoephedrine are found in cold preparations. They are useful in reducing nasal congestion and opening up the airways to your lungs.)

However, these over-the-counter drugs and the herbal preparation ephedra should not be used by patients with heart and vessel disease. These drugs and herbal preparations increase heart rate and elevate blood pressure. Some people abuse ephedra, taking high doses for long periods of time to increase alertness or to lose weight. Higher doses of ephedra can lead to amphetamine-like side effects, such as high blood pressure, rapid heartbeat or palpitations, nervousness, irritability, headache, difficulty urinating, vomiting, insomnia, and even heart attack, heart failure, or sudden death.

Chinese black licorice (glycyrrhizic acid is the active ingredient) is used primarily as a flavoring for some herbal preparations. However, it should be avoided by heart patients because it can cause life-threatening arrhythmias. Chinese licorice contains an ingredient that makes your body excrete potassium. Potassium levels can become very low, causing the heart to beat erratically.

St. John's wort is an herbal supplement that may benefit people with mild depression. However, it also activates an enzyme in the liver that breaks down many medicines. By accelerating the breakdown of medicines, St. John's wort can interfere with the effectiveness of some drugs. For example, it may interfere with the ability of Coumadin to thin the blood. If you are a heart disease patient taking Coumadin, you should not use St. John's wort. St. John's wort has also been known to trigger rejection in people with heart transplants. If you have heart disease and are on medication, you should check with your doctor before using St. John's wort.

IS THIS SUPPLEMENT WORKING FOR ME?
A METHOD OF SELF-EVALUATION

Try one supplement at a time and use the evaluation process outlined below to help determine how well it is working. When you find one that works, you don't need to try any others. If you are only experiencing partial benefit, you could test a combination of supplements, again using the method outlined below to determine efficacy.

Try each supplement for about one to three months.

If you are taking a supplement for chest pain or shortness of breath due to a heart problem, you should note whether you are having less discomfort with the same amount of activity. Keep a "Symptom Diary," in which you note the following:

- Time and duration of any chest pain or shortness of breath and what you were doing at the time. Note how severe the pain was (on a scale from 1 to 10, where 1 is no pain and 10 is the most severe pain).

- If you are taking medicine intermittently for episodes of pain (for example, a tablet of nitroglycerin to stop an episode of chest pain), note how often you had to take the medicine during the day.

- Record how well you did during your daily exercise program. How far did you walk without developing chest pain or shortness of breath?

- Keep the diary for at least one month before and at least one to three months during your use of the new supplement.

- Take a close look at the diary for those months. Determine if you were able to exercise longer without pain or shortness of breath. Add up how many times you had pain or shortness of breath during the day or night. If your symptoms have not been reduced in number or severity, and if you have not had an improvement in your exercise tolerance, you may want to stop using the supplement; it may not be doing you any good. Talk to your doctor about the lack of improvement in your symptoms; the doctor may recommend that you stop that supplement.

- *Remember that the supplement does not replace the drugs your doctor has prescribed.*

If you are taking a supplement for leg pain while walking, you should determine whether the nutritional therapy is reducing your leg pain.

- Keep a "Walking Diary," in which you note your walking distance each day.

- Keep the diary for at least one month before and at least one month (preferably two months) after starting the nutritional supplements.

- *Remember that the supplement does not replace the drugs your doctor has prescribed.*

If you are taking a supplement for pain or swelling in the legs (due to problems with your veins or lymphatics), then determine if the supplement is helping.

- One way to determine how much swelling you have is to put a tape measure around your calf at its midpoint and measure the circumference of your leg. (You need to note exactly where you measured so that you can take the measurement in the same spot each time.)

- Take the measurement weekly to determine if the swelling has decreased.

- Also note how often and how severe the leg pain is before and during use of the supplement.

If you are taking a supplement to lower cholesterol

- Have your doctor check your cholesterol before and after you have been on the nutritional therapy for two months.

If you are taking a supplement to lower blood pressure

- Have your blood pressure checked several times a week for one month before and during use of the supplement.

If you are taking a supplement to regulate blood sugar

- Have your doctor check your blood sugar and glycHb (glycosylated hemoglobin) before and after you have been on the therapy for one month.

Yohimbine, which increases blood pressure and heart rate, should not be taken by heart patients.

A number of other supplements are known to thin the blood and can therefore increase the effect of blood thinners given to you by your doctor. If you are taking Coumadin, check with your doctor before taking any new supplements.

Chapter 11

Already Ill–Intensive Care
for Your Blood Vessels

THE ADVICE in this chapter applies to men who scored 6 to 10 (or over 10) and women who scored 11 to 15 (or over 15) on the Point System Risk Assessment in Chapter 7. Your endothelium is severely impaired and you are at risk for a heart attack or stroke. What do you need to know to prolong your life and restore the health of your blood vessels? This chapter will give you information you need to feel better and extend your life. Think of this chapter as arming yourself. Once you read it, you will be better able to help your doctor stop, and even reverse, the progression of your vascular disease.

Warning Signs and Symptoms of Heart Disease

YOUR SCORE indicates that you have lost your self-defense mechanism against atherosclerosis. You have an increased risk of having a heart attack or stroke in the future, particularly if you are a man over the age of 40 or a woman over the age of 50. For this reason, it is important that you know the signs and symptoms of heart disease. They are there for a reason. They are a signal from your body that it is in distress.

Symptoms occur when blood flow is reduced by narrowings in the arteries. Blood flow reduction can occur in different parts of the body, resulting in heart disease, stroke, peripheral arterial disease, or in some cases, more than one of these diseases.

If you have any of the warning signs, *your score on The Point System Risk Assessment is an underestimate of your risk*. You already have advanced hardening of your arteries and should see a physician immediately. These warnings should be taken very seriously, particularly if you have several risk factors. These warning signs may indicate that you are about to have a heart attack or a stroke. If you have several risk factors but don't have these symptoms, it doesn't mean you are free and clear. Unfortunately, for about half the people who have heart disease, the first symptom is a heart attack. The same is true of carotid artery disease. Your first symptom could be a stroke. By taking The Point System Risk Assessment, and by paying attention to the warning signs, you have a better chance of protecting yourself.

Heart Disease or Heart Attack

AS I'VE explained, some people have no warning signs of heart disease at all. Others have angina, the term used to describe the feeling of discomfort in the chest caused by reduced blood flow to the heart arteries.

You may experience angina as one or more of the following:

- uncomfortable pressure, fullness, squeezing, or pain in the center of the chest lasting more than a few minutes
- indigestion or a "burning" in the chest
- discomfort in the chest that spreads to the shoulders, neck, or arms
- chest discomfort with light-headedness, fainting, sweating, nausea, or shortness of breath
- chest discomfort with a choking feeling or a feeling of tightness in the throat

I've seen a handful of individuals with heart disease who have decidedly unusual symptoms. They complain of

- discomfort in the left arm
- discomfort in either shoulder

· discomfort between the shoulder blades
· discomfort in the left jaw

In most people, the tip-off that this pain is a warning sign for heart disease (and not indigestion, for example) is that the symptoms come on during physical exertion, mental stress, or after eating a heavy meal. If the discomfort comes on during exertion, it may come on faster if you are rushing, going up a hill, or if it is cold outside.

Stable angina is a condition in which a person has angina of the same severity for several months or years. The angina is triggered in a similar manner every day by the same activities—for example, walking up three flights of stairs, or shoveling snow, or emotional stress. The angina is relieved a few minutes after resting or taking a nitroglycerin tablet.

Unstable angina is a condition in which the angina suddenly becomes much worse. The severity and duration of pain may be greater. Or it takes much less activity to bring on the discomfort. Or it may take more rest and/or more nitroglycerin to relieve the pain. By definition, angina that occurs for the first time is unstable angina.

If you have unstable angina, immediately call your doctor. You may be getting close to having a heart attack. You may need to have your medication increased and have some additional testing done. Your doctor may want to perform an EKG and check some blood tests immediately.

If you have had angina for years but one day your symptoms persist for more than 10 minutes and are not relieved by nitroglycerin, you may be in serious trouble and should contact a physician. Persistent discomfort for more than 20 minutes (unrelieved by nitroglycerin) is characteristic of a heart attack. Immediately call your doctor, 911, or have someone drive you to the emergency room. If you have nitroglycerin, place a tablet under your tongue (or if you have a nitroglycerin spray, spray some onto your tongue). Also, chew and swallow an aspirin. Taking aspirin during the early stages of a heart attack has been shown to reduce death and disability from a heart attack, especially when combined with early medical treatment.

A heart attack is often accompanied by shortness of breath, sweating, extreme fatigue, and sometimes a sense of impending doom. Men often deny their symptoms. They pass off the pain as indigestion and don't tell anyone until the discomfort is severe. Even then, it is often their wives who force them to go to the emergency room. If you are having symptoms similar to those described above, it is not the time for silent stoicism.

It is important to act quickly, because 50 percent of people who have a heart attack die before they reach the hospital. This is tragic because we now have blood-clot-busting drugs and catheter procedures that can open up a blocked artery and prevent damage to the heart during an attack.

Realize too that not everyone who has angina is doomed to have a heart attack. Some people live with intermittent, but stable, angina for years. If you follow my program for endothelial health, your angina may never develop into a heart attack and your symptoms may subside.

Carotid Artery Disease or Stroke

THERE ARE also warning signs for stroke or carotid artery disease. The carotid arteries in the neck supply the brain with blood. A stroke is caused when plaque in the carotid artery ruptures, causing clot and plaque debris to go to the brain.

If this happens, you may experience:

- a sudden weakness or numbness of the face or in an arm or leg on one side of the body
- loss of speech, difficulty communicating, or trouble in understanding speech
- sudden dimness or loss of vision, particularly the feeling that a shade is being pulled down over one eye
- unexplained dizziness, unsteadiness, or sudden falls, especially along with any of the above symptoms

Often, these symptoms subside quickly, over a period of minutes. Called a TIA (transient ischemic attack), the sudden onset of symptoms is a warning sign that should be taken very seriously. Immediately call your doctor, 911, or have someone drive you to the emergency room. There are now clot-busting medicines and procedures that can prevent stroke or reduce the severity of a stroke in progress.

The milder the stroke, the easier it is to recover. Some people recover from a small stroke with only mild weakness or numbness in an arm or a leg, slight difficulty speaking, and occasionally with no obvious problem at all. By contrast, people who have a major stroke may lose the ability to speak or comprehend, or may not be able to move one side of the body.

Peripheral Arterial Disease (PAD)

PAD, HARDENING of the arteries in the leg vessels, is one of the most underdiagnosed diseases of the blood vessels. In the 1999 PAD Awareness, Risk, and Treatment: New Resources for Survival (PART-NERS) study, about 10,000 people were screened for PAD with blood pressure measurements of the legs. Of those, about 25 percent over the age of 70 had PAD; and about 25 percent of people over the age of 55 with diabetes or a history of smoking had PAD. The most worrisome finding of the study? Only a third of the patients' doctors knew they had PAD. The rest had the condition, but their doctors were not aware of it. This is worrisome, because people with PAD are at a greatly increased risk of heart attack and stroke.

Many people have symptoms of PAD without knowing that they have a circulation problem. They attribute their leg discomfort to the aches and pains of growing old. But the symptoms of PAD are recognizable if you know what to look for. When the vessels supplying blood to the legs narrow, the first signs are:

- cramping, fatigue, heaviness, or aching of the buttocks, thighs, or calves while walking
- leg pain that comes on faster if you are walking up a hill, carrying a heavy load, or walking quickly
- aching of the foot, worse at night, relieved by dangling the foot over the bed or standing up
- leg pain that goes away when you stand still or rest

PAD is a disease that is frequently overlooked by doctors. Many have not been trained in the diagnosis of PAD and may think that it is a benign disease (as long as you don't have severe pain or gangrene) and that there is not much that can be done medically to treat it. It is important for you or your physician to recognize the symptoms of PAD because it is not benign. If you have PAD, you are much more likely to have silent narrowings in the heart arteries (silent because you can't walk far enough or quickly enough to have angina).

You are also more likely to have carotid artery disease and are at risk for stroke. The leg vessel disease may also be accompanied by impotence.

PAD patients should be cared for by a physician who carefully monitors the disease. Your doctor should put you on an exercise program (after first evaluating you during a treadmill test). There are some dietary supplements that may help. (See Chapter 10.) I generally recommend aspirin or another antiplatelet medication; you may also need medication to lower cholesterol and blood pressure. We now have specific medicines, such as cilostazol, that relieve PAD symptoms. On average, this medication can increase walking distance by about 50 percent.

Occasionally, pain in the leg may come on suddenly because of sudden blockage of a leg vessel by a clot (either because a clot has broken off of the aorta or heart and floated downstream to block a leg artery or because one of the leg arteries has a plaque that has ruptured and clotted off the leg artery). In this case, you will feel severe and persistent leg and foot pain, and your foot will be pale, cool, and numb. Any of these warning signs should immediately alert you to seek the advice of a doctor.

IF PAD GETS WORSE . . .

Without proper diet, exercise, risk reduction, supplementation, and medication, PAD can get worse. Here are some symptoms that may indicate this:

- pain that sets in very quickly when walking
- healing of cuts and wounds that takes longer
- no hair growth on legs
- toes that become dark red
- black or dark spots or ulcers that appear at the tips of the toes, heels, or ankles

When symptoms worsen, it may be necessary to consult with a vascular specialist. An angiogram may be recommended to determine whether the condition can continue to be treated medically or if angioplasty or bypass surgery is necessary.

Testing for Plaque in the Vessels

HOW CAN you tell if you have plaque? Knowing how many risk factors you have helps. The more you have, the more likely that you have plaque. If you have several risk factors, and if you are a man over 40 or a woman over 50, it is reasonable to have some tests to determine if you have significant hardening of the arteries. Following are some of the most common tests used to detect vessel disease.

TEST FOR PAD

What is it: Ankle-brachial index.

Why: The test compares blood pressure at the ankle and arm. The two measurements should be the same. If blood pressure at the ankle is less, then you have hardening of the arteries in your legs. (The blood pressure is less because the narrowings in the leg arteries reduce the flow of blood and the pressure transmitted to the vessels.) It is also likely that you have significant deposits in your heart and carotid arteries.

Who needs it: Everyone over the age of 70, and anyone who experiences cramping, fatigue, or heaviness of the buttocks, thighs, or calves while walking. People over the age of 55 who have diabetes or who smoke. (If symptoms don't respond to medical treatment, additional tests such as ultrasound of the leg arteries or angiography may be necessary.)

TEST FOR CAROTID ARTERIES (STROKE)

What is it: Ultrasound of the carotid arteries.

Why: Ultrasound is very good at detecting plaque in the carotid arteries. It provides an image of the artery, much as ultrasound can provide an image of a baby during a prenatal exam.

Who needs it: Everyone who is at high risk (see The Point System Risk Assessment, p. 182), particularly if they have a bruit, a noise in the neck like a murmur that can be heard with a stethoscope. The bruit is caused by turbulent flow in the carotid artery due to a narrowing or twisting of an artery. Also, anyone who has symptoms suggestive of a transient ischemic attack (described on p. 238).

Tests for Heart Disease

THERE ARE a variety of tests used to diagnose damage to the heart and narrowing of the heart arteries. Sometimes patients may require more than one test.

EKG OR ELECTROCARDIOGRAM

What is it: An EKG records the flow of electricity through your heart. Electrodes are attached to the skin on your chest and a machine prints out a display of each beat of your heart (which starts with an electrical impulse). By looking at the readout, a physician can see any changes in the way your heart is beating.

Why: An EKG can identify a variety of problems. It can tell if the heart is enlarged, showing signs of strain, or has abnormal rhythms. It can detect thickening in the heart muscle, faulty conduction of electrical signals, areas of scarring due to a prior heart attack, and evidence of poor blood flow to the heart.

Who needs it: Everyone over 40, particularly if they have risk factors for heart disease or if they need to have any type of major surgery (which would place a strain on the heart).

STRESS TEST

What is it: Stress tests are examinations performed while you exercise to determine if your heart is getting enough oxygen or whether narrowings in your heart arteries are limiting blood flow. A stress test can be done several ways. The simplest way is to monitor the EKG while you walk on a treadmill. If your coronary arteries are narrowed, your heart will not get enough blood flow to meet the increased demands of exercise, and your EKG will show specific changes reflecting the strain on your heart.

There are other, even more sensitive ways of taking pictures of the heart during exercise. Echo stress testing uses ultrasound to create a picture of the heart at work. From this test, we can see how well the heart is pumping during exercise and determine whether valves are leaking or if the walls of the heart are thickened.

During yet another method, radionuclide stress testing, patients receive an intravenous injection of a small amount of radioactive tracer. Because the tracer is carried by the blood, the physician sees less tracer in those parts of the heart that are not getting enough blood flow. During exercise, a special camera is used to detect the tracer and to see which areas of the heart are receiving adequate blood flow. If a patient has trouble walking and can't perform an exercise test, medication can be given intravenously to challenge the heart. The patient is then given an echo or radionuclide study before and after the medication is given.

Why: Stress tests are performed to determine if areas of the heart are not getting enough blood flow when the heart is challenged.

Who needs it: Anyone at high risk should have a treadmill exercise test. If you are at moderate risk and about to embark on a new exercise program, have major surgery, or some other physically stressful event in your life, you should have a treadmill exercise test. The echo or radionuclide tests are a little more accurate and provide some additional information that may be useful to your doctor.

HEARTSCAN

What is it: HeartScan is a noninvasive test that is purported to detect plaque. It measures the amount of calcium in your heart vessels, which is believed to be correlated to the amount of plaque. (Generally the more plaque you have, the more calcium you have in your coronary arteries.)

Why: When a person develops atherosclerosis in the heart arteries, there is often some calcium present in the plaque. When we use microscopes to look at plaque, we often see small areas of calcification. Intriguingly, in the microscope, these small areas in the blood vessel are virtually indistinguishable from bone (which is composed of bone protein and calcium). It turns out that there are cells in the vessel wall that can produce bone protein that then becomes calcified. These bony deposits can also occur in plaque.

This observation has led some researchers to suggest that bony deposits in the vessel wall could be markers for hardening of the arteries. This has led to the development of machines, such as the HeartScan, that provide images of calcium in the vessel wall. The HeartScan uses electron beam computed tomography (EBCT) to detect calcium in the heart and coronary arteries.

Who needs it: We do not yet have enough information about whether this type of test is more useful than evaluating standard risk factors in determining risk of heart attack. I have some doubts about it. If you have your cholesterol, blood sugar, and blood pressure checked, these risk factors, along with your family history, can predict your chance of having a heart attack possibly as well as the HeartScan (and at significantly less cost). In one evaluation at the Harbor-UCLA Medical Center, about 1,200 Californians with risk factors for heart disease had both standard risk-factor evaluation and EBCT scanning. They were then closely monitored for more than three years. The researchers found that EBCT was no better than evaluating the standard risk factors for predicting who would have a heart attack.

However, when people see a picture of calcium in their heart arteries, they may be more likely to stick to the recommendations of their doctor.

ANGIOGRAPHY

What is it: Angiography or angiogram is known as the "gold standard" in detecting narrowings in the blood vessels. It is considered an invasive test since it requires a puncture into one of your blood vessels. In most cases, patients are first given local anesthesia. Then a thin tube is passed through a hollow needle into the leg or arm artery. The tube is pushed into position just at the point where the heart arteries branch off the aorta. The physician inserts a catheter through the tube and threads it up through the artery that branches off the aorta.

At this point, a liquid dye that can be seen by X ray is infused into the catheter. In this way, the cardiologist can see whether an artery is narrowed or blocked.

Why: This test can help the cardiologist and surgeon determine if narrowings in the heart arteries can be repaired by angioplasty or surgery. (See p. 257 for my comments about angioplasty.)

Who needs it: Patients with severe or unstable angina. Patients who are having a heart attack. An angiogram is always a prerequisite for angioplasty. Patients who have stable angina or abnormal results on a stress test or echocardiogram may also need an angiogram. (For people who have stable angina, I recommend the test only to those who have tried and failed to reduce their symptoms with diet, exercise, supplementation, and medication.) Of note, an angiogram does have a small risk associated it. About 1 in 1,000 angiograms are complicated by a potentially life-threatening event: bleeding from the puncture site (where the catheter enters the artery); reaction to the liquid dye; or heart attack or stroke (if the catheter knocks off a plaque from the aorta or its branches).

Unfortunately, there are no noninvasive tests that can provide clear images of the coronary arteries. Echocardiography cannot detect plaque in the coronary arteries because the air in the lungs interferes with the images. One day soon, magnetic resonance imaging may be used.

INTRAVASCULAR ULTRASOUND

What is it: Intravascular ultrasound, a new technique for imaging coronary plaque, can determine the size of the plaque and provide information about its characteristics (how much calcium, how much fat, how much scar tissue). A catheter bearing a small ultrasound transducer is placed inside the coronary artery to get information about the lumen and the wall of the vessel.

Why: It is a technique that provides even more detail than angiography.

Who needs it: Intravascular ultrasound has become particularly useful for determining if stents are placed properly in the coronary artery. It is also useful for patients who have had heart transplants, because angiography in these cases can miss significant narrowings.

Test for Endothelial Function

ENDOTHELIAL FUNCTION TEST

What is it: Endothelial function testing is an exciting new and noninvasive approach to assessing the health of blood vessels. This approach is largely used at research centers and is not yet widely available. However, it will be. I predict that in the next five years, this test will become as common as, and at least as important as, blood pressure measurements.

Why: Now that we know more about blood vessel and endothelial function, we know how important they are to overall vascular health.

There are several ways to assess endothelial function; most involve testing the endothelium's ability to relax the vessel wall or to make the vessel wall more compliant. At Stanford, we use ultrasound to test endothelial function. By imaging the arm arteries, we can see how well they respond to increases in blood flow.

The test is easy and noninvasive. Here's how it works: When blood flow increases through a vessel with a healthy endothelium, the vessel opens up wider to accommodate the increase. You can see this flow-mediated vasodilation, as it's called, by using ultrasound. First we increase blood flow through the arm. We do this by placing a blood pressure cuff around the wrist and inflate it to a pressure high enough to cut off blood flow to the hand. After five minutes, we release the cuff and the blood rushes back into the hand. This sudden increase in blood flow stimulates the endothelium to make NO, and in response, the arm artery increases in diameter for a short period of time. We can see the vessel dilate by using an ultrasound device. We know how well your endothelium is functioning by how much your arm artery dilates.

When a patient has an unhealthy endothelium, we try different lifestyle, nutritional, and medication adjustments. The patient then returns in a few weeks; we perform the ultrasound test again to see if blood vessel health has improved.

I am convinced that a noninvasive and rapid test of endothelial function will become widespread for several reasons:

• It immediately indicates the health of your blood vessels.

· Through repeat tests, we can determine whether lifestyle, nutrition, supplements, or medication changes are improving vessel health, and your medical program can be tailored to your specific needs.

· Most important, this test can predict your risk of having a heart attack or stroke. In fact, several studies indicate that endothelial function may be a better predictor for heart attack and stroke than all others.

Who needs it: When a simple noninvasive endothelial test is more widely available, I will recommend it for everyone over the age of 40 and everyone under the age of 40 with risk factors. Children who have risk factors might also benefit from this test.

Treating Cardiovascular Disease

INTENSIVE CARE FOR YOUR VESSELS

AS YOU know, if you are a man who scored 6 to 10 (or over 10) or a woman who scored 11 to 15 (or over 15) on The Point System Risk Assessment in Chapter 7, you need intensive care for your vessels. If you have any of the signs and symptoms of heart and vessel disease discussed above, the intensity of the care increases further. First, you need to begin my diet. You need to start an exercise program *after* you have had a treadmill test to make sure that you can exercise safely. And, most likely, you will need some of the supplements described in Chapter 10, tailored to your specific risk factors and symptoms. It is also likely that you will need one or more of the medications described below. Your physician can guide you in the selection of the right supplements and medications for your condition. The following information will be useful to you in this process.

DRUGS THAT WORK

ONCE YOU'VE been tested for heart disease and your physician understands the intricacies of your heart health, he or she may prescribe a variety of different medications.

I've seen many patients turn away from medications in hopes that a particular diet or supplement will save them. Many diet books and health gurus may try to convince you that you can avoid drug therapy by following a specific diet. While it's true that a healthy diet and lifestyle are critical parts of preventive medicine, diet gurus do a tremendous disservice to heart patients by maintaining that a specific diet can replace all drug therapy. If you are a heart patient, don't believe this propaganda. If you have heart disease, your body very likely needs additional support. Most of the dietary regimens or health foods recommended by these self-proclaimed experts have not undergone the same kind of rigorous clinical trials that medications have as part of the FDA approval process.

People also resist taking medication because they prefer natural remedies. I understand this reluctance. It is based on a reasonable belief that a natural approach is best. Indeed, our bodies are highly evolved, with a great complexity that is only just beginning to be understood by medical science. I also lean toward understanding and enhancing the body's natural mechanisms for self-healing. However, there are situations where these natural mechanisms for self-healing need greater support. The best strategy is diet, exercise, supplements, and/or medications that are tailored to your needs by a doctor who is knowledgeable in blending natural and pharmacological approaches for heart health. The best strategy is one that integrates all of the therapies that can restore the normal function of your heart and blood vessels.

If you already have heart disease, or are at high risk, there are medical therapies that can support and restore these natural mechanisms and can save your life. Studies show that, unfortunately, many people who could benefit from these medical therapies are not taking them. In some cases, this is because doctors are not always aware of clinical trials that show the benefits of a particular drug. Or they are not aware that their patient is at high risk and needs medication to reduce that risk. In addition, many HMOs do not put enough emphasis on good preventive care, nor do they pay doctors to take the time to dispense this type of care.

If you have any type of vascular disease, you should be taking one or more of the following drugs. If you do not have heart disease but are at high risk, you may also benefit from one or more of these medications.

Following are the most common medications for vascular disease and what you need to know about them. Talk to your doctor about them.

Aspirin

Description: Antiplatelet medication. Although aspirin itself does not improve endothelial function, it does prevent clots from forming as a result of abnormal endothelial function.

Use: Individuals taking aspirin are 20 to 30 percent less likely to have a heart attack or stroke.

Dose: There is some controversy about how much aspirin people need. Sir John Vane, the Nobel laureate who discovered how aspirin works, was frequently asked how much aspirin one should take. His advice? "Take one aspirin out of your medicine chest. Lick it. Put it back. Tomorrow, take another lick." Obviously Sir John thought that low-dose aspirin was sufficient.

On the other hand, some doctors recommend higher doses (up to three adult aspirins daily) because some people are resistant to lower doses of aspirin (they still form blood clots in their vessels).

Side effects: There are risks with high-dose aspirin, including stomach ulcers and bleeding. Higher doses may suppress the ability of the blood vessels to make prostacyclin, a natural protective factor. However, the benefits of aspirin in any dose outweigh the risks.

Similar medications: Clopidogrel, a new antiplatelet medicine, is as safe as aspirin, although more expensive. A recent study of about 20,000 people with heart and vessel disease showed that in these people, clopidogrel was slightly superior to one adult aspirin daily in reducing heart attack, stroke, and death from vascular disease.

My recommendation:

- If you are a man or woman older than 40 and have risk factors for heart disease, you should take at least 81 milligrams (one baby aspirin) daily (unless your physician tells you otherwise).
- If you are at high risk, you should take one adult aspirin daily.
- If you have had a heart attack or stroke, particularly if you were on aspirin at the time, ask your doctor about clopidogrel.

Beta-Blockers

Description: Beta-blockers, such as propranolol, slow down the heart rate and reduce blood pressure—and basically reduce the work of the heart. These drugs are designed to block the effect of adrenaline (which makes the heart beat faster and harder). In animals with high cholesterol levels, beta-blockers improve endothelial function and slow the progression of atherosclerosis.

Use: Beta-blockers are excellent drugs to reduce blood pressure, relieve angina, lessen palpitations, and decrease the chances of a second heart attack or death.

Side effects: The major side effect from beta-blockers is feeling physically and/or mentally slowed down, even depressed. Beta-blockers have been associated with impotence. They have a slight adverse effect on blood lipids and a tendency to raise cholesterol. Nevertheless, there are many studies showing that this drug saves lives, specifically in people who have had a heart attack or those who have a weak heart. Many people take this drug with minimal or no side effects. (In people who have diabetes, beta-blockers should be used under strict supervision since they can reduce the body's ability to respond to an episode of insulin-induced hypoglycemia, a very low blood sugar due to too much insulin. Hypoglycemia can cause damage to your heart and brain if it is not corrected quickly.)

My recommendation: Beta-blockers should be considered as a first-choice therapy for people with angina, particularly those who have had a heart attack. They are a good treatment for high blood pressure and for irregular heartbeats. They are also helpful for patients with heart failure (most doctors don't recommend them often enough for this condition). For people with heart failure, they should be started at low doses and carefully increased. The beta-blocker carvedilol is a particularly good choice for patients with heart failure.

Because beta-blockers may slow people down, I sometimes recommend an ACE inhibitor rather than a beta-blocker to reduce blood pressure in hypertensive people who have not had a heart attack.

ACE Inhibitors

Description: Vasodilator. ACE (angiotensin-converting enzyme) inhibitors prevent the production of angiotensin II (AII), a hormone produced by the kidneys and blood vessels. AII causes blood vessels to contract, thereby reducing blood flow and increasing blood pressure. ACE inhibitors block the enzyme in the body that makes angiotensin II, and breaks down the body's vasodilator, bradykinin. ACE inhibitors also increase the release of NO from the vessels and reduce the blood vessels' production of free radicals that can destroy NO.

Use: By reducing the production of AII, ACE inhibitors reduce blood pressure, improve blood flow, and make the work of the heart easier. They improve endothelial health and can be used to treat hypertension and to relieve angina. In animals, ACE inhibitors have been found to prevent atherosclerosis, mainly because they improve NO production and activity.

ACE inhibitors improve the survival of people with heart disease, particularly those who have had a heart attack and those with weak hearts (reduced pumping function of the heart, also known as heart failure). By reducing blood pressure, the ACE inhibitors reduce the work of the heart. By resting the heart in this way, its pumping function can improve over time.

There are some ACE inhibitors that may be better at enhancing NO release than others. These tissue-specific ACE inhibitors reportedly get into the blood vessel wall better than other ACE inhibitors. For this reason, these drugs seem to be better at enhancing the release and activity of NO.

ACE inhibitors can be used with beta-blockers or in place of beta-blockers to reduce blood pressure and the work of the heart.

Side effects: Although rare, the most frequent side effects are dry cough, bad taste in the mouth, and light-headedness (from blood pressure that is too low).

Similar medications: A new class of drugs, known as angiotensin receptor blockers (ARBs), is similar to the class of ACE inhibitors. ARBs have very few side effects and are just as effective as ACE inhibitors in reducing blood pressure. They can also improve endothelial function. However, because they are new, there have not been as many studies with these drugs and there is less evidence they prevent heart disease and extend life.

My recommendation: ACE inhibitors enhance endothelial health. If you have hypertension, an ACE inhibitor is an excellent drug to lower your blood pressure. I also strongly recommend it for people with heart failure. If you are over the age of 55 and have diabetes or vessel disease (but not high blood pressure or heart failure), ACE inhibitors could prevent you from having a heart attack or stroke. If you have had a heart attack and/or if your heart is weak, you should ask your doctor why you are not on an ACE inhibitor. If the ACE inhibitor causes a side effect that you can't tolerate, one of the ARBs may be a reasonable alternative.

ACE inhibitors are also particularly good for people with diabetes. They reduce the risk of heart attack and stroke by about 30 percent in people with diabetes; they also preserve kidney function. There is even evidence that ACE inhibitors can reduce the risk of developing diabetes.

Diuretics

Description: Also known as water pills, diuretics are drugs that increase the kidneys' excretion of water and salt. This reduces the volume of blood that the heart needs to pump, and by lessening the heart's work, lowers blood pressure.

Use: Diuretics are inexpensive and effective drugs that have been used for a long time to lower blood pressure and to help in the treatment of heart failure. The thiazide diuretics (such as hydrochlorothiazide, or HCTZ) have been shown (when used by themselves or with other blood pressure medications) to reduce stroke and heart attack in people over the age of 60 with high systolic blood pressure (pressure over 160). In people over the age of 60 with high systolic pressure, the addition of a calcium channel blocker to the diuretic regimen may be necessary to gain control of blood pressure.

It is important to get systolic blood pressure down to 140 and the diastolic pressure down to 80 (no matter what medication is being used). Unfortunately, in the United States, fewer than one-quarter of patients who have high blood pressure are receiving effective treatment.

Side effects: These diuretics can cause gout in a small percentage of patients. They can also slightly increase cholesterol levels and reduce potassium levels. You may need potassium supplementation if you are taking these pills.

My recommendation: If you have heart failure, these water pills are quite helpful in combination with ACE inhibitors. I also recommend them for patients over 60 with high blood pressure, often in combination with a vasodilator, such as an angiotensin-converting enzyme inhibitor (ACEI).

Statins

Description: Cholesterol-lowering drugs.

Use: Since their introduction in the 1980s, statins have become the most potent cholesterol-lowering medicines that we have today. Statins are designed to inhibit an enzyme known as HMG-CoA reductase that is needed in the production of cholesterol. When the statins block HMG-CoA reductase, the liver can't make cholesterol. But the liver cells need a certain amount of cholesterol to form cell membranes and to function properly. Since the liver cells can't make cholesterol, they need to get it from somewhere else. So they get their cholesterol from the blood, by producing receptors that collect LDL (bad) cholesterol. This leaves less bad cholesterol floating around and accumulating in the bloodstream.

Statins also work in other ways. They directly increase the amount of NO synthase in the vessel wall. By increasing NO production, statins reduce inflammation of the blood vessel and markers for inflammation in the bloodstream.

Statins also stabilize plaque and prevent it from rupturing. (They don't necessarily reduce the size of the plaque, although over a period of several years there may be a slight reduction in plaque size.) The stabilization process includes an improvement in endothelial function (with an increase in NO activity), which returns the endothelium to its Teflon-like state. Statins work quickly too; within weeks, they can improve endothelial function in people with high cholesterol. Statins also rapidly improve endothelial function in people who have had a recent heart attack.

By reducing cholesterol and enhancing endothelial function,

statins save lives. Both pravastatin and simvastatin have been shown to reduce heart attack, stroke, and death in people who are at risk for heart and vessel disease. In terms of lowering cholesterol, the most potent of the statins is atorvastatin, which can reduce cholesterol levels by 30 to 40 percent. A similar benefit can be achieved with other statins at higher doses. (Statins can also lower cholesterol with the help of drugs that bind cholesterol in the intestines so that it is excreted. These are the bile-acid-binding resins such as cholestyramine and colesevelam.)

Statins are very good at lowering LDL cholesterol, but much less effective at raising HDL cholesterol. Niacin is somewhat better in this regard.

Side effects: Liver function should be carefully monitored. Occasionally, the statins (like all antilipid medications) can cause a chemical hepatitis that resolves rapidly if the problem is noticed and the medicine is withdrawn. Rarely, statins cause muscle damage or inflammation (myositis) that is manifested by persistent muscle aches and weakness and increased blood levels of a muscle enzyme. This also subsides when the medication is stopped. (One statin, cerivastatin, was pulled off the market in 2001 because it was responsible for severe myositis, causing death in a number of people.)

Similar medications: Gemfibrozil is another drug that can raise HDL cholesterol and is also particularly good at reducing triglycerides. Recent evidence from a trial carried out at the Veterans Administration hospitals revealed that gemfibrozil could increase HDL cholesterol by about 6 percent. This increase in HDL cholesterol was associated with a 22 percent reduction in death or disability from heart disease.

Fibrates, niacin, and bile-acid binders are also effective at lowering cholesterol, but they are not as powerful as statins. There is not as much data on the use of these drugs, as compared to statins, regarding their long-term effects on the risk of heart attack, stroke, and death.

My recommendation:

- If you are otherwise healthy with no risk factors for heart disease other than high cholesterol, first try my diet and exercise program. If your total cholesterol remains over 200 (and particularly if your LDL cholesterol is over 160), then try some of the cholesterol-lowering nutritional supplements. If your cholesterol remains at unsatisfactory levels, talk to your doctor about a lipid-lowering medicine such as a statin.

• If you have high cholesterol as well as other risk factors but no symptoms of heart and vessel disease, start on my diet, exercise, and nutritional supplement program. Depending on how many risk factors you have, your doctor may wish to start you on medicine right away to get your LDL cholesterol under 130.

• If you have high cholesterol and symptoms associated with narrowed vessels, you will need to see your doctor about cholesterol-lowering medicine. That is because the levels of cholesterol that are safe for you are much lower than those that are safe for a healthy person with no risk factors. Your doctor should try to get your LDL cholesterol below 100 and your HDL cholesterol above 45.

If medicine is needed to lower LDL cholesterol, then statins are my favorite, mainly because the data show that they powerfully lower LDL cholesterol—and save lives. If it is necessary to further reduce LDL cholesterol, or to raise HDL cholesterol, statins can be used in combination with niacin. In addition, the daily use of a stanol ester–containing margarine improves the effect of statins, further lowering your cholesterol. If the main problem is low HDL cholesterol, niacin can be very helpful in raising it (together with daily exercise and one serving daily of wine or another alcoholic beverage). If the natural approach is not completely successful, then the drug gemfibrozil may be a useful addition.

Spironolactone

Description: Reduces excessive accumulation of fluid and salt in the body.

Use: You won't hear much about this medicine because it is now generic.[1] It is very helpful for a weak heart (heart failure) and may prevent fibrosis (scar formation) within the blood vessels and heart. Fibrosis causes vessels and heart tissue to become stiffer. When your heart and vessels are stiffer, the work of the heart is increased, requiring more energy to pump blood through the vessels. If your heart is already weak, it doesn't need to do more work, and fibrosis could cause your heart to fail faster. A recent clinical trial, the Randomized Aldactone Evaluation Study (RALES), showed that the addition of spironolactone to the regimen of people with heart failure reduced their risk of death from heart failure by 30 percent.

Side effects: Spironolactone can cause men to develop enlargement and tenderness of the breasts, a side effect that disappears when the drug is stopped.

My recommendation: If you have heart failure, you should probably be taking this drug. However, it has to be used cautiously and in lower doses when combined with ACE inhibitors, because the combination could increase the potassium in your blood to dangerous levels.

MEDICATIONS THAT I GENERALLY AVOID

Calcium Channel Blockers (Short-Acting)

Description: Short-acting calcium channel blockers are very effective at reducing blood pressure—in fact, too effective. They lower blood pressure so quickly that you actually feel faint. The rapid drop in blood pressure can cause an increase in heart rate that strains your heart and may even trigger a heart attack.

Today, there are better calcium channel blockers that are longer acting and that cause a more gradual and longer-lasting drop in blood pressure, with less heart rate increase. These are useful drugs to lower blood pressure and to relieve chest pain. However, they are not as effective as beta-blockers and ACE inhibitors for preventing heart attack, so in my opinion they are a third choice in the treatment of hypertension and angina.

Nitrates (Long-Acting)

Description: Long-acting nitrates, such as nitroglycerin patches and oral preparations, are used to treat angina. They work because they release NO or because they contain NO as part of their structure. In a sense, they are a replacement for NO. Unfortunately, though, when you administer these nitrates for a long time, the body makes less NO on its own. Over time, these nitrates actually impair the ability of the endothelium to relax the blood vessel. It is even possible that this drug-induced impairment of the endothelium can accelerate hardening of the arteries. Indeed, there is evidence from animal models that suggests that long-term administration of oral nitrates can hasten atherosclerosis.

The lesson from these observations is that our endothelium is smarter than the pharmaceutical industry. NO is a potent molecule, and it is made by the endothelium as needed, in the amounts needed, and where needed. The production of NO occurs in response to physiological stimuli. Activating these natural physiological stimuli—through diet, supplements, and exercise—is all the body needs to help it make its own supply of NO.

My advice: Short-acting nitroglycerin tablets or oral sprays are excellent ways to relieve angina during painful episodes. However, I avoid oral and topical long-acting nitrate preparations. Instead, I help people improve their body's ability to make NO so that they don't need even the short-acting nitroglycerin.

THE PROS AND CONS OF SURGERY

"My Doctor Says I Need an Angioplasty"—Read This First

Every year in this country, about 900,000 angioplasties, the procedure to open up narrowed blood vessels, are performed to treat arteries that have narrowed or are blocked by plaque. If the narrowing is in a heart artery, the procedure involves a balloon catheter (a hollow tube with a small inflatable balloon on its end) inserted through an arm or leg artery and pushed up into the heart artery. The catheter is placed into the narrowed segment so that the balloon is at the site of blockage. The balloon is inflated and the heart artery is opened up. (Over 500,000 heart angioplasties are performed every year; the rest are performed in the leg, kidney, or other arteries.)

Angioplasty is an expensive procedure, costing between $5,000 and $20,000, depending on where it is performed, how many vessels are opened, and how many stents are used. It is a procedure often recommended for patients with chronic angina that doesn't respond to medication.

In a minority of these angioplasty cases, there is a clear and compelling reason to perform the procedure. In the middle of a heart attack, it is important to get to the hospital immediately and to receive blood-thinning medicine, angiography, clot-busting drugs, and/or angioplasty. This aggressive and interventional approach saves lives in the middle of a heart attack. But if a person has stable symptoms, there is time for nutritional and medical therapy in an attempt to allow the body to heal itself.

I recommend that patients have angioplasty only if their symptoms are not well controlled by medical and nutritional therapy, or if their stress test becomes particularly worrisome. But I am cautious about recommending this procedure. Not all narrowings of the arteries need to be opened up by a catheter. Most of the time, they can be treated by nutritional and lifestyle changes and a good medical program. Unfortunately, many cardiologists tend to have an "oculodilator reflex"—they see a narrowing and they automatically dilate it (with a catheter).

Here are some of the pros and cons of the procedure, as I see them. We used to believe that angioplasty worked because the balloon simply compressed the plaque that was narrowing the coronary artery. By compressing the plaque, we believed the blockage would be reduced at that site. But we now know that this view was simplistic. What actually happens is this: As the balloon inflates, the plaque cracks and the vessel wall tears. The vessel opens up, but it is severely damaged at the site of the balloon inflation. The endothelium is ripped off the vessel at the site of the angioplasty. This damage causes clotting to occur, which is usually prevented by giving patients anticoagulants (blood thinners) and antiplatelet drugs at the time of the procedure. In 1 out of 200 cases, the vessel is immediately obstructed by clot and the angioplasty fails. When this happens, or when the balloon inflation has not sufficiently opened up the vessel, another procedure is used—this time involving a stent, a small metal coil that can expand, placed at the site of obstruction.

The stent is placed over the balloon of the catheter. As before, the catheter is placed into the heart artery and the balloon (covered by the stent) is placed into the narrowed region. The balloon is then inflated, and the stent expands. When the balloon is deflated, the catheter is withdrawn with the stent left behind, holding the vessel open.

Using both techniques, angioplasty is successful in 98 to 99 percent of cases. Opening up the heart artery improves blood flow and relieves chest pain. So it would seem that angioplasty is a worthwhile procedure.

But there is one big problem with successful angioplasties. Angioplasty is a form of controlled trauma to the vessel. Through the process of opening the vessel through angioplasty, the vessel itself becomes injured. The body then tries to repair this damage. A scar forms—made from connective tissue and the smooth muscle cells in the coat of the injured vessel wall—and moves into the injured area. In some angioplasty patients, the scar formation is excessive, the vessel again narrows, and the chest pain recurs. This process of re-narrowing is called restenosis. In 40 percent of cases, there is a chance that the artery will re-narrow after the procedure. Restenosis is reduced to about 20 percent with stents. Most drugs, given orally to prevent restenosis, fail. Often, doctors attempt a second or third angioplasty to try to remedy the problem. All of these invasive procedures increase the risk of a life-threatening complication, not to mention boosting medical costs.

Restenosis is an animal unlike any other. Whereas atherosclerosis takes decades to narrow a vessel, restenosis takes a much shorter time—about three to six months. We have many drug and nutritional therapies to treat atherosclerosis, but most of our drugs seem to fail with restenosis. (Recent data suggest that the drugs probucol or cilostazol, used for PAD, may help reduce restenosis. Unfortunately, probucol is no longer available in the U.S. because of its potential to cause irregular heart rhythms, and cilostazol can increase heart rate, which is not good for heart patients.) Ironically, in an attempt to help blocked arteries through angioplasty, cardiologists often replace atherosclerosis (a disease that can be treated) with restenosis (a disease that is less responsive to medical therapy). Although the use of stents has reduced restenosis to about 10 to 20 percent of cases, stents do not completely prevent restenosis because the smooth muscle cells can grow in between the coils of the stent.

Restenosis will be less of a problem in the future when new drug-releasing stents are approved by the FDA. Also some cardiologists are now using radiation to prevent restenosis—with some success. In this procedure, a special catheter filled with a radioactive substance is threaded up into the heart arteries, exposing the segment where the balloon or stent was placed to radiation for a few minutes. Then the radioactive catheter is withdrawn from the heart arteries. Too much radiation can irreversibly damage the vessel wall and cause an aneurysm (like a bulge in a tire, this is a weak and thinned point in the vessel wall that expands outward and can rupture). In addition, the long-term consequences of this radiation treatment are unknown. For these reasons, once an effective drug is approved by the

FDA, radiation therapy for restenosis will disappear. Even so, whereas angioplasty and stenting can relieve symptoms, these expensive procedures do not treat the disease process. It is far better to make nutritional and lifestyle changes, and when necessary take supplements and medications, to prevent vessel disease in the first place. When a patient has symptoms, I advise a full-court press with medical therapy before going to expensive and invasive interventions. In those people who need angioplasty and a stent, I also advise a sustained and aggressive nutritional and medical program to prevent atherosclerosis from striking again.

WHEN ANGIOPLASTY DOESN'T WORK

While the majority of angioplasties are successful and relieve symptoms, 1 to 2 percent of patients don't end up with an opened vessel after the procedure. For these people, several risks can crop up and, in some cases, cause life-threatening complications.

In about 1 percent of angioplasties, the procedure is complicated by life-threatening problems at the time of the procedure. Some vessels simply don't respond, or clot off during the procedure. The patient may then require emergency open-heart bypass surgery. In some patients, heavy bleeding may occur at the leg artery, the artery typically punctured by the cardiologist to get to the blood vessels. The puncture site may open up, and a significant amount of blood can be lost. Although there are special devices and medications that can be used to prevent bleeding at the puncture site, internal bleeding can still occur if a vessel is accidentally punctured as the catheter is placed up the leg artery into the aorta and the heart arteries.

Similarly, when the cardiologist threads the catheter up the aorta toward the heart, the catheter may push up against a plaque and break it. This can cause clotting to occur near the plaque. If it happens in the heart artery, it can cause a heart attack. In the aorta, bits and pieces of plaque and clot can break off and go anywhere in the body. Debris in the leg arteries can block the foot arteries, causing the toes to become blue and painful ("trash foot syndrome"). If the debris gets into the kidney arteries, it can cause kidney failure. (I know several patients who had to go on dialysis after an angiographic procedure knocked debris into their kidney arteries.) Debris that enters the arteries in the stomach can cause abdominal pain and even destroy a portion of the intestines. Plaque that enters the neck arteries can result in stroke.

Still other patients have a reaction to the drugs and contrast agents (substances that can be seen on X ray) used during the procedure. These substances are placed into fluids infused into the heart arteries as an X ray is taken. The cardiologist can then see the heart arteries and tell where they have narrowed. A small percentage of the population has an allergic reaction to the contrast agent. (If you are allergic to shellfish or to iodine-containing substances, you are more likely to have a reaction.) Sometimes the reaction is mild (hives or an itchy rash, usually on the trunk, arms, and legs), but sometimes it can be more worrisome (swelling of the face, shortness of breath) or even life-threatening (a serious drop in blood pressure, inability to breathe).

Is Surgery Worth the Risk?

It's important to remember that angioplasty can reduce the symptoms of heart disease but not the disease itself. Even those patients who have a successful angioplasty are not free of disease.

Angioplasty is a surgical solution to the problems of blocked arteries, but it does not address the cause of the narrowing—atherosclerosis. After angioplasty, patients are still at risk for heart attack or stroke from a plaque somewhere else in the vessel.

Angioplasty does not generally save lives (except for those people saved while in the middle of a heart attack). But it is effective at relieving the symptoms of chest pain. And in patients who have not responded to diet, exercise, and medication, it is a very useful procedure to relieve pain. However, it should not be attempted when patients have stable angina—and all nutritional and medical approaches have not been tried. There are medications as well as nutritional approaches that can relieve chest pain at less cost and less risk. Furthermore, these drug therapies and nutritional approaches have been shown in the long term to reduce risk from heart attack and stroke (whereas angioplasty has not).

With the huge cost and number of risks involved in this procedure, surely there must be some data that show that angioplasty is superior to medical therapy? I am sorry to report that there is not. Coronary angioplasty can relieve symptoms, but there is no evidence that it saves more lives than medical therapy. And the bulk of the data indicate that bypass surgery is more effective than angioplasty at reducing pain, keeping people out of the hospital, and generally keeping them alive longer.

For all of these reasons, I view angioplasty as a treatment of last resort. I have seen too many patients with serious complications from angioplasty that could have been avoided. Unfortunately, many cardiologists feel differently. Many of my colleagues are too quick to draw this arrow out of their quiver. In my opinion, about half of the angioplasties performed in this country are unnecessary. There are occasions, however, when coronary angioplasty is useful, usually in emergency situations or when medical and nutritional therapy fails.

I send very few patients to the cardiac cath lab for angioplasty. It has been my experience that an endothelial health program— with nutrition and lifestyle changes, together with medication as needed—is almost always sufficient to relieve angina. My approach has been supported by a large clinical study conducted in 1999, the Atorvastatin Versus Revascularization Treatment (AVERT) trial. In this study, 341 patients with mild to moderate angina who were scheduled for angioplasty were allowed to proceed with angioplasty or were placed on an aggressive lipid-lowering regimen (a low-cholesterol diet and the statin atorvastatin). Patients were then monitored for a year and a half. In patients on the aggressive lipid-lowering regimen, LDL cholesterol went down to 80. For those who had angioplasty, LDL cholesterol went down to 120. In the people who took aggressive lipid-lowering drugs, there were fewer heart problems than in those who had angioplasty (as well as a 36 percent reduction in surgeries, procedures, and hospitalizations). This study suggests that aggressive medical therapy is superior to angioplasty. In my opinion, it is far better, and well within your ability, to restore the health of your endothelium rather than have a cardiologist remove it with a balloon catheter. If your doctor recommends angioplasty, tell him or her that if at all possible, you prefer a medical and dietary approach. Angioplasty should be reserved for emergency situations (when someone is in the middle of a heart attack) or when medical and nutritional therapy have been attempted but failed to relieve the symptoms.

If your doctor still insists that you need angioplasty or surgery for your heart and vessel disease, get a second opinion, preferably from a cardiologist who does not perform invasive procedures.

As for bypass surgery, there was a time in the 1970s when bypass surgery was believed to be superior to medical therapy if a patient had three major vessels that were diseased or had disease of the left main coronary artery (the vessel that gives rise to two of the major heart arteries). However these are old data. The difference between surgical and medical therapy in terms of their effect on quality and quantity of life has narrowed. Medical therapy has improved considerably since then, with whole new classes of drugs that were not available in the 1970s. Our understanding of vessels, vessel disease, and how to reverse the disease process has increased dramatically.

In my opinion, medical and nutritional therapy should be the first line of treatment for all patients with heart and vessel disease. In people whose symptoms have failed aggressive medical and nutritional therapy, including supplements, angioplasty may be reasonable. Bypass surgery is a better choice for those patients who have three diseased vessels or left main coronary artery disease, particularly if the heart is not pumping as well as it should.

NO AND RESTENOSIS

Restenosis is due in part to the growth and multiplication of vascular smooth muscle cells in the vessel wall. NO can prevent smooth muscle cells from growing and multiplying. In animal studies, we have found that inserting the gene for NO synthase into the vessel wall at the time of angioplasty increases NO production for a sustained period of time—and this is associated with a reduction in restenosis. My research team and others have observed the same benefit by infusing the vessel wall with L-arginine or proteins composed of L-arginine. These animal studies have launched studies in humans to determine if restenosis can be averted by increasing NO production in the vessel wall.

Chapter 12

On the Road to a Healthy Endothelium

UNTIL NOW, patients and physicians have found out about the endothelial health program via word of mouth. Here is one of my favorite examples. Dr. Joseph Kozina, a well-respected and busy cardiologist in Sacramento, California, sits on the board of the local affiliate of the American Heart Association (AHA). I met him when I was invited to speak to the board about the AHA-funded research that I had carried out at Stanford. (The AHA has provided us with several grants to investigate hardening of the arteries and the role of NO in making vessels healthy.)

Dr. Kozina was intrigued by the research, and we had a nice conversation about the implications of the work. Sometime later, Dr. Kozina saw a patient, Ms. Mildred Mineau, in his office. Mildred had a long history of heart disease and had undergone bypass surgery years before. Now she was back in Dr. Kozina's office, complaining of an increase in the frequency and severity of her chest pain. An angiogram ruled out any possibility for repeat bypass surgery or angioplasty. (Some patients are too frail or their vessels are too diseased for repeat surgery or angioplasty.) Already on maximum medical therapy, Mildred was having 12 to 15 episodes of angina daily. Just trying to do housework brought on chest pain.

Then Dr. Kozina remembered his conversation with me. He introduced Mildred to the medical food that I had developed to improve endothelial function. Within a couple of weeks Mildred began to notice a profound reduction in her symptoms. When she returned to see Dr. Kozina, she thanked him profusely for introducing her to this new strategy for heart health. Dr. Kozina was delighted to hear that the frequency and severity of Mildred's pain was markedly better, down to about one or two episodes of angina a day and easily relieved by a nitroglycerin tablet. Mildred was so pleased with her improved condition that she called the medical food a "magical meal" because of the remarkable difference it made in her life.

My research in endothelial health satisfies my curiosity about understanding how healthy blood vessels function. But my work is even more gratifying and exciting when the research is applied to people—and it improves their health. For me, there is no greater achievement than improving the lives of patients through research.

I hope that you are as encouraged as I am by this new research in NO. We now know that you are only as old as your endothelium. And, fortunately, you can restore the health of your endothelium, heart, and vessels with dietary measures and exercise. The health of your endothelium is in your hands. You can, and should, take the first steps toward a healthier and longer life.

Good luck on the road to a healthy endothelium and a lifetime of cardiovascular health! If you follow the recommendations in this book, you will restore and enhance your natural defense against heart disease and stroke. Take the steps necessary to activate your body's natural defense against cardiovascular disease.

Along the way, if you need more help, please feel free to visit my website at www.cardiovascularcure.com. The field of cardiovascular medicine, nutrition, and endothelial health is developing quickly. New therapies are on the horizon, as are new technologies to assess endothelial function. These developments will help us in our quest for the cardiovascular cure, a healthy endothelium.

What is this C-reactive protein (CRP) that I'm hearing so much about right now?

CRP is a blood protein that is part of the body's inflammatory response. CRP levels are high in those with infectious or inflammatory disease, but they are also elevated in those at risk for heart disease. CRP might be a new method to test risk for cardiovascular disease.

What do I do if my doctor doesn't know anything about endothelial health?

There is increasing awareness in the medical community about the importance of endothelial health. This book has useful information in it for physicians and provides references where they can get additional information. (See Information for Your Doctor, p. 271.)

What does NO have to do with an aneurysm?

An aneurysm is a weak and thinned point in the vessel wall in the brain that expands outward and can rupture like the blowout of a tire. Aneurysms are more likely to form in people who have atherosclerosis (hardening of the arteries). Atherosclerosis occurs in people who have an unhealthy endothelium. NO made by the endothelium prevents processes that lead to hardening of the arteries. Recently a direct link was made between NO and aneurysms. Dr. Paul Huang and colleagues in Boston removed the gene for endothelial NO synthase in mice with high cholesterol. These mice, whose endothelium could not make NO, developed aneurysms and tears in the aorta. The mice who could make NO did not have this complication.

Is there a relationship between a herpes infection and heart disease?

There is some indirect evidence that herpes virus, cytomegalovirus, chlamydia, or other infectious agents could accelerate hardening of the arteries. These infectious agents, which have been found in plaque, are known to trigger the inflammation involved in plaque formation. People who have been infected by these germs have a greater chance of having coronary artery disease. However, it has not been proven that in humans these germs accelerate atherosclerosis, nor has it been shown that treatment of these infections will prevent or slow hardening of the arteries.

Is L-arginine the solution for heart disease?

There is no one solution for the prevention of symptoms of heart and vascular disease. Most people just need to follow the dietary and exercise recommendations that I have outlined in this book. Others may also benefit from supplements (such as L-arginine), or need medication or even surgery. This book provides some guidance about what measures you can take to restore the health of your endothelium. However, this book is not a replacement for the advice of your health professional, particularly if you have heart disease.

Do you lose your endothelial lining with heart disease?

Not until very late stages, and only then in small areas. Even if you have advanced heart or vessel disease, you can still enhance the health of your endothelium.

How will the endothelial health program help me if I already have heart disease?

If you already have heart disease, your endothelium is not healthy. It is already like Velcro; platelets and white blood cells stick and accumulate, causing plaque to grow. Inflammation of the plaque is more likely to occur if your endothelium is unhealthy, and this could lead to plaque rupture and a heart attack. It is important for you to restore the health of your endothelium to avoid a heart attack or stroke.

What does it mean when the heart becomes enlarged?

When the heart has been exposed to high blood pressure and/or stiff vessels for a long time, it can begin to wear out. Although the heart continues to beat normally, the walls of the heart thicken. As time goes on, the heart may begin to increase in size and doesn't contract as well. This is one cause of heart enlargement and heart failure. It can also become enlarged and pump poorly after a viral infection affecting the heart. When the valves of the heart leak and/or become narrowed, this increases the work of the heart and can lead to thickening of the heart wall and enlargement of the heart.

What is beating-heart surgery?

When surgeons operate on the heart to put in bypass grafts around occluded vessels, they usually stop the heart so that it is easier to work on. During the time the heart is stopped, a machine pumps blood throughout the body. However, as blood travels through the machine, small clots can form on the artificial surfaces of the machine, and these small clots can be circulated throughout the body, even into the brain. To avoid these problems, surgeons are beginning to use a beating-heart approach. When the chest is opened up, the heart is allowed to continue to beat naturally (a machine is not used to pump the blood). To operate on the beating heart, surgeons use special clamps and tools to steady the area of the heart on which they are operating.

Is there a limit on how much aerobic exercise is good for your endothelium? Does more than 30 minutes a day make your endothelium healthier?

There is some evidence that greater intensity and duration of exercise can provide even more benefit for your blood vessels. For example, Dr. Bill Haskell at Stanford has shown that middle-aged ultramarathoners have coronary arteries that can relax much better than those of couch potatoes, with a maximum increase in caliber that is twice as great. However, moderate exercise (a 30-minute brisk walk daily) will be easier for most people to do over the long term.

If the endothelium is so important, why haven't I heard about it until now?

The biology of the endothelium is one of the hottest areas in cardiovascular science today. Several Nobel Prizes have been awarded for discoveries linked to the endothelium—most recently in 1998, to the three American scientists who discovered endothelium-derived nitric oxide. However, it takes years, sometimes decades, for the best science to be translated into something useful.

What is dysfunctional endothelium?

When your endothelium is healthy, it is like Teflon; the blood flows smoothly through the vessel. The healthy endothelium keeps the vessel relaxed, wide open, and pliable. However, risk factors such as high cholesterol make the endothelium dysfunctional. The dysfunctional endothelium is more like Velcro. Cells begin to stick and enter into the vessel. Also, the vessel is more likely to constrict or spasm and limit blood flow. The vessel is still lined by endothelium, but the endothelium is not working properly.

How does a healthier endothelium affect arrhythmias, atrial fibrillation, or other heart problems related to electrical charge?

The most common cause of arrhythmias in this country is high blood pressure. Another common cause is coronary artery disease. If you have a healthy endothelium, your blood pressure will be lower. If you have a healthy endothelium, you will not get coronary artery disease.

Until now, cholesterol seemed to be most important to cardiovascular health. Now that we know about the endothelium, which is more important, cholesterol level or endothelial health?

Endothelial health is the cardiovascular cure. Cholesterol is important, and you should definitely follow the guidelines laid out in this book regarding healthy cholesterol levels. But cholesterol is just one risk factor of many that can impair the health of the endothelium.

If it is true that atherosclerosis can begin to develop in children, what can parents do to ward off the beginnings of this disease?

Nutrition and exercise. Children need to eat more fruit, vegetables, nuts, legumes, and fish. They need to eat less fried food and fast food. They need to get more exercise. If heart disease occurs at an early age in the family, talk to your child's physician. Your child may need some blood tests to determine risk.

Can a glass of wine really help your endothelium?

Wine in moderation is good for your endothelium. One or two drinks daily with meals is beneficial to your heart and vessels. However, you can get a similar benefit from eating a bunch of fresh grapes, which is a distinctly better approach if you have trouble drinking alcohol in moderation.

Why is a healthy endothelium the cardiovascular cure?

The healthy endothelium keeps your vessels open and your circulation flowing. The healthy endothelium makes substances that protect your vessels, like nitric oxide (NO). The healthy endothelium is like a Teflon lining for your vessel, preventing cells from sticking and preventing plaque from forming.

Information for Your Doctor

Information for Your Doctor about the Endothelium and Nitric Oxide

In the last decade, there has been a logarithmic growth of knowledge in vascular biology. We have learned much about the determinants of vascular reactivity and structure. A proliferation of cell surface and nuclear receptors have been characterized, as have a multiplicity of signal transduction and transcriptional pathways that are activated with ligand-receptor interactions. A host of vasoactive mediators have also been found to regulate the growth of vascular cells and their interaction with blood elements. The endothelium plays a critical role in vascular homeostasis by virtue of the paracrine substances that it elaborates. One of the most active of these endothelium-derived factors is nitric oxide (NO). NO is a potent vasodilator that also inhibits platelet aggregation, prevents leukocyte adherence and infiltration, and suppresses the proliferation and migration of vascular smooth muscle cells. In this way, NO is an endogenous antiatherogenic agent.

References:

Berk, B.C. 2001. Vascular smooth muscle growth: Autocrine growth mechanisms. *Physiol Rev* 81(3)(July): 999–1030.

Candipan, R.G., et al. 1996. Regression or progression: Dependency upon vascular nitric oxide. *Arterioscler Thromb Vasc Biology.* 16(1)(January): 44–50.

Cooke, J.P., et. al. 2001. Nitric oxide and vascular disease. In *Nitric Oxide: Biology and Pathobiology*. Edited by Louis Ignarro. San Diego: Academic Press.

Cooke, J.P., and V.J. Dzau. 1997. Nitric oxide synthase: Role in the genesis of vascular disease. *Annu Rev Med* 48: 489–509.

Hickey, M.J., and P. Kubes. 1997. Role of nitric oxide in regulation of leuco-cyte-endothelial cell interactions. *Exp Physiol* 82(2)(March): 339–48.

Ignarro, L.J., et al. 2001. Role of the arginine-nitric oxide pathway in the regulation of vascular smooth muscle cell proliferation. *Proc Natl Acad Sci USA* 98(7)(27 March): 4202–8.

Loscalzo, J. 2001. Nitric oxide insufficiency, platelet activation, and arterial thrombosis. *Circ Res* 88(8)(27 April): 756–62.

Murad, F. 1999. Discovery of some of the biological effects of nitric oxide and its role in cell signaling. *Bioscience Reports* 19(3): 133–54.

Information for Your Doctor about ADMA

ADMA is asymmetrical dimethylarginine, an endogenous antagonist of NO synthase. ADMA is derived from the normal breakdown of protein in the course of cell catabolism. It is excreted in the urine and becomes markedly elevated in patients with renal failure, contributing to the severe endothelial dysfunction observed in these patients. ADMA is also broken down by the enzyme DDAH (dimethylarginine dimethylaminohydrolase). In patients with risk factors, ADMA is elevated, due to oxidative impairment of DDAH. The elevation in ADMA appears to correlate better with endothelial dysfunction than does LDL cholesterol in hypercholesterolemic subjects.

References:

Boger, R., et al. 1998. Asymmetric dimethylarginine (ADMA): a novel risk factor for endothelial dysfunction: its role in hypercholesterolemia. *Circulation* 98(18)(3 November): 1842–47.

Chan, J.R., et al. 2000. Asymmetric dimethylarginine increases mononuclear cell adhesiveness in hypercholesterolemic humans. *Arterioscler Thromb Vasc Biol* 20(4)(April): 1040–46.

Cooke, J.P. 2001. Does ADMA cause endothelial dysfunction? *Arterioscl Thromb Vasc Biol* 20(9)(September): 2032–37.

Ito, A., et al. 1999. Novel Mechanism for Endothelial Dysfunction: Dysregulation of Dimethylarginine Dimethylaminohydrolase. *Circulation* 99(24)(22 June): 3092–95.

Miyazaki, H. et al. 1999. Endogenous nitric oxide synthase inhibitor: a novel marker of atherosclerosis. *Circulation* 99(9)(9 March): 1141–46.

Vallance, P., et al. 1992. Accumulation of an endogenous inhibitor of nitric oxide synthesis in chronic renal failure. *Lancet* 339(8793)(7 March): 572–75.

Information for Your Doctor about Atherosclerosis and the Endothelium

Accumulating data indicate that atherosclerosis begins and ends with endothelial dysfunction. Impairment of endothelial function leads to monocyte adherence and infiltration and formation of the fatty streak. With loss of endothelial health, the lesion grows as vascular smooth muscle, and in-flammatory cells migrate into the lesion and proliferate. Endothelial dys-function also contributes to the terminal event, plaque rupture, which is due to inflammation of the plaque. Thus, endothelial dysfunction increases the risk of a cardiovascular event. Therefore, at all stages of atherosclerosis, restoration of endothelial function can improve cardiovascular health.

References:

Celermajer, D.S., et al. 1994. Endothelium-dependent dilation in the sys-temic arteries of asymptomatic subjects relates to coronary risk factors and their interaction. *J Am Coll Cardiol* (24)(6)(15 November): 1468–74.

Fuster, V., Z.A. Fayad, and J.J. Badimon. 1999. Acute coronary syndromes: bi-ology. *Lancet* 353(June)Suppl 2:SII5–9.

Ghiadoni, L., et al. 2000. Mental stress induces transient endothelial dys-function in humans. *Circulation* 102(20)(14 November): 2473–78.

Griendling, K.K., and D.G. Harrison. 2001. Out, damned dot: studies of the NAD(P)H oxidase in atherosclerosis. *J Clin Invest* 108(10)(November): 1423–24.

Heitzer, T., et al. 2001. Endothelial dysfunction, oxidative stress, and risk of cardiovascular events in patients with coronary artery disease. *Circula-tion* 104(22)(27 November): 2673–78.

Libby, P. 2001. Current concepts of the pathogenesis of the acute coronary syndromes *Circulation* 104(3)(17 July): 365–67.

Ludmer, P.L., et al. 1986. Paradoxical vasoconstriction induced by acetyl-choline in atherosclerotic coronary arteries. *N Engl J Med* 315(17)23 Oc-tober): 1046–51.

Navab, M., et al. 1996. The yin and yang of oxidation in the development of the fatty streak. A review based on the 1994 George Lyman Duff Memor-ial Lecture. *Arterioscler Thromb Vasc Biol* 16(7)(July): 831–42.

Oemar, B.S. et al. 1998. Reduced endothelial nitric oxide synthase expres-sion and production in human atherosclerosis. *Circulation* 97(25)(30 June): 2494–98.

Ross, R. 1999. Atherosclerosis—an inflammatory disease. *N Engl J Med* 340(2)(14 January): 115–26.

Schachinger, V., M.B. Britten, and A.M. Zeiher. 2000. Prognostic impact of coronary vasodilator dysfunction on adverse long-term outcome of coro-nary heart disease. *Circulation* 101(16)(25 April): 1899–906.

Suwaidi, J.W., et al. 2000. Long-term follow-up of patients with mild coro-nary artery disease and endothelial dysfunction. *Circulation* 101(9)(7 March): 948–54.

Information for Your Doctor about Nutrition and the Endothelium

What you eat has a dramatic effect on the health of your endothelium. Within hours of eating a high-fat or methionine-enriched diet (typical West-ern diet), endothelial function becomes impaired. By contrast, a number of nutritional substances can enhance vascular function, including antioxidant vitamins; L-arginine (see below); soy protein and phytoestrogens; and omega-3 fatty acids. What you eat has acute effects on the ability of the blood vessel to relax, and in the long term, will have dramatic effects on the structure of the blood vessel.

References:

Cuevas, A.M. et al. 2000. A high-fat diet induces and red wine counteracts endothelial dysfunction in human volunteers. *Lipids* 35(2)(February): 143–48.

Dillinger, T.L., et al. 2000. Food of the Gods: Cure for Humanity? A cultural history of the medicinal and ritual use of chocolate. *The Journal of Nutrition.* 130(85)(August): 20575–715.

Duffy, S.J., et al. 2001. Short- and long-term black tea consumption reverses endothelial dysfunction in patients with coronary artery disease. *Circulation* 104(2)(10 July): 151–56.

Fard, A., et al. 2000. Acute elevations of plasma asymmetric dimethylarginine and impaired endothelial function in response to a high-fat meal in patients with type 2 diabetes. *Arterioscler Thromb Vasc Biol* 20(9)(September): 2039–44.

Fitzpatrick, D.F., et al. 1993. Endothelium-dependent vasorelaxing activity of wine and other grape products. *Am J Physiol* 265(2 Pt 2)(August): H774–78.

Lissin, L., and J.P. Cooke. 2000. Phytoestrogens and their effects on the cardiovascular system. *J Am Coll Cardiol* 35(6)(May): 1403–10.

Plotnick, G.D., M.C. Corretti, and R.A. Vogel. 1997. Effect of antioxidant vitamins on the transient impairment of endothelium-dependent brachial artery vasoactivity following a single high-fat meal. *JAMA* 278(20)(26 November): 1682–86.

Stein, J.H., et al. 1999. Purple grape juice improves endothelial function and reduces the susceptibility of LDL cholesterol to oxidation in patients with coronary artery disease. *Circulation* 100(10)(7 September): 1050–55.

Stühlinger, M.C., et al. 2001. Homocysteine impairs the NO synthase pathway—Role of ADMA. *Circulation* 104(21)(20 November): 2569–75.

Tagawa, H., et al. 1999. Long-term treatment with eicosapentaenoic acid augments both nitric oxide-mediated and non-nitric oxide-mediated endothelium-dependent forearm vasodilatation in patients with coronary artery disease. *J Cardiovasc Pharmacol* 33(4)(April): 633–40.

Timimi, F.K., et al. 1998. Vitamin C improves endothelium-dependent vasodilation in patients with insulin-dependent diabetes mellitus. *J Am Coll Cardiol* 31(3)(1 March): 552–57.

Vogel, R.A., M.C. Corretti, and G.D. Plotnick. 2000. The postprandial effect of components of the Mediterranean diet on endothelial function. *J Am Coll Cardiol* 36(5)(1 November): 1455–60.

Information for Your Doctor about Nutrition, Exercise, and Cardiovascular Events

Accumulating evidence indicates that about one-third of cardiovascular deaths can be prevented by proper exercise and nutrition. Exercise enhances endothelial function and prevents progression of atherosclerosis. Nutritional interventions that are consistent with endothelial health also prevent cardiovascular events.

References:

Ajani, U.A., et al. 2000. Alcohol Consumption and Risk of Coronary Heart Disease by Diabetes Status. *Circulation* 102: 500.

Appel, L.J., et al. 1997. A clinical trial of the effects of dietary patterns on blood pressure. *N Engl J Med* 336: 1117–24.

de Lorgeril, M., et al. 1999. Mediterranean diet, traditional risk factors, and the rate of cardiovascular complications after myocardial infarction: Final report of the Lyon Diet Heart Study. *Circulation* 99(6)(16 February): 779–85.

Detrano, R.C., et al. 1999. Coronary calcium does not accurately predict near-term future coronary events in high-risk adults. *Circulation* 99(20)(25 May): 2633–38.

Fitzpatrick, D.F., et al. 1995. Endothelium-dependent vasorelaxation caused by various plant extracts. *J Cardiovasc Pharmacol* 26(1)(July): 90–95.

Fraser, G.E., et al. 1992. A possible protective effect of nut consumption on risk of coronary heart disease. The Adventist Health Study. *Arch Intern Med* 152(7)(July): 1416–24.

Grundy, S.M., et al. 1999. Assessment of Cardiovascular Risk by Use of Multiple-Risk-Factor Assessment Equations. *Circulation* 100: 1481–92.

Hambrecht, R., et al. 2000. Effect of exercise on coronary endothelial function in patients with coronary artery disease. *N Engl J Med* 342(7)(17 Feb): 454–60.

Hambrecht, R. et al. 1998. Regular physical exercise corrects endothelial dysfunction and improves exercise capacity in patients with chronic heart failure. *Circulation* 98(24)(15 December): 2709–15.

Haskell, W.L., et al. 1994. Effects of intensive multiple risk factor reduction on coronary atherosclerosis and clinical cardiac events in men and women with coronary artery disease. The Stanford Coronary Risk Intervention Project (SCRIP). *Circulation* 89(3)(March): 975–90.

Hiatt, W.R., et al. 1996. Effect of exercise training on skeletal muscle histology and metabolism in peripheral arterial disease. *J Appl Physiol* 81(2)(August): 780–88.

Hornig, B., V. Maier, and H. Drexler. 1996. Physical training improves endothelial function in patients with chronic heart failure. *Circulation* 93(2)(15 January): 210–14.

Hu, F.B., and M.J. Stempfer. 1999. Nut consumption and risk of coronary heart disease: a review of epidemiologic evidence. *Curr Atheroscler Rep* 1(3)(November): 204–9.

Imhof, A., et al. 2001. Effect of alcohol consumption on systemic markers of inflammation. *Lancet* 357(9258)(10 March): 763–67.

Jacobs. D.R., et al. 2001. Reduced mortality among whole grain bread eaters in men and women in the Norwegian County Study. *Eur J Clin Nutr* 55(2)(February): 137–43.

Kris-Etherton, P., et al. 2001. AHA Science Advisory: Lyon Diet Heart Study. Benefits of a Mediterranean-style, National Cholesterol Education Program/American Heart Association Step I Dietary Pattern on Cardiovascular Disease. *Circulation* 103(13)(3 April): 1823–25.

Lee, I.M., et al. 2001. Physical activity and coronary heart disease in women: is "no pain, no gain" passe? *JAMA* 285(11)(21 March): 1447–54.

Moroney, J.T., et al. 1999. Low-density lipoprotein cholesterol and the risk of dementia with stroke. *JAMA* 282(3)(21 July): 254–60.

Niebauer, J., and J.P. Cooke. 1996. Cardiovascular effects of exercise: Role of endothelial shear stress. *J Am Coll Cardiol* 28: 1652–60.

Oomen, C.M., et al. 2001. Association between trans fatty acid intake and 10-year risk of coronary heart disease in the Zutphen Elderly Study: a prospective population-based study. *Lancet* 357(9258)(10 March): 746–51.

Sacks, F.M., et al. 2001. Effects on blood pressure of reduced dietary sodium and the Dietary Approaches to Stop Hypertension (DASH) diet. DASH-Sodium Collaborative Research Group. *N Engl J Med* 344(1)(4 January): 3–10.

Schachinger, V., et al. 2000. Prognostic impact of coronary vasodilator dysfunction on adverse long-term outcome of coronary heart disease. *Circulation* 101(16)(25 April): 1899–906.

Taddei, S., et al. 2000. Physical activity prevents age-related impairment in nitric oxide availability in elderly athletes. *Circulation* 101(25)(27 June): 2896–901.

Vogel, R.A., M.C. Corretti, and G.D. Plotnick. 2000. The postprandial effect of components of the Mediterranean diet on endothelial function. *J Am Coll Cardiol* 36(5)(1 November): 1455–56.

Information for Your Doctor about Risk Factors and Endothelial Function

Endothelial dysfunction is the common pathway by which all risk factors cause atherosclerosis. Endothelial dysfunction causes abnormal vascular reactivity in the short term and pathological changes in vascular structure in the long term. All of the traditional risk factors are known to induce endothelial dysfunction. The dysfunctional endothelium can be detected long before any observable changes in the vessel wall. Abnormal endothelial function is the first detectable vascular abnormality in response to risk factors and is a prerequisite for the development of atherosclerosis.

Medications that improve endothelial function also reduce cardiovascular events. Most notable in this regard are the statins and the angiotensin-converting enzyme inhibitors. Statins improve endothelial function by reducing LDL cholesterol, but they also have some direct effects on the NO synthase pathway (specifically they increase the expression and/or activity of NO synthase in the vessel wall). Angiotensin-converting enzyme inhibitors reduce the breakdown of bradykinin, and by so doing, increase NO synthase activity. Furthermore, ACE inhibitors decrease angiotensin II–induced production of superoxide anion (which degrades nitric oxide). By so doing, ACE inhibitors prolong the action of nitric oxide. Other drugs that enhance endothelial function may also prove to reduce cardiovascular events.

References:

Anderson, T.J., et al. 1995. The effect of cholesterol-lowering and antioxidant therapy on endothelium-dependent coronary vasomotion. *N Engl J Med* 332(8)(23 February): 488–93.

Balletshofer, B.M., et al. 2000. Endothelial dysfunction is detectable in young normotensive first-degree relatives of subjects with type 2 diabetes in association with insulin resistance. *Circulation* 101(15)(18 April): 1780–84.

Celermajer, D.S., et al. 1992. Non-invasive detection of endothelial dysfunction in children and adults at risk of atherosclerosis. *Lancet* 340(8828)(7 November): 1111–15.

Creager, M.A., et al. 1990. Impaired vasodilation of forearm resistance vessels in hypercholesterolemic humans. *J Clin Invest* 86: 228–34.

Mancini, G.B., et al. 1996. Angiotensin-converting enzyme inhibition with quinapril improves endothelial vasomotor dysfunction in patients with coronary artery disease. The TREND (Trial on Reversing Endothelial Dysfunction) Study. *Circulation* 94(3)(1 August): 258–65.

Panza, J.A., et al. 1990. Abnormal endothelium-dependent vascular relaxation in patients with essential hypertension. *N Engl J Med* 323(1)(5 July): 22–27.

Schachinger, V., et al. 1999. A positive family history of premature coronary artery disease is associated with impaired endothelium-dependent coronary blood flow regulation. *Circulation* 100(14)(5 October): 1502–8.

Sessa, W.C. 2001. Can modulation of endothelial nitric oxide synthase explain the vasculoprotective actions of statins? *Trends Mol Med* 7(5)(May): 189–91.

Information for Your Doctor about Drugs, Endothelial Function, and Cardiovascular Events

Farquharson, C.A., and A.D. Struthers. 2000. Spironolactone increases nitric oxide bioactivity, improves endothelial vasodilator dysfunction, and suppresses vascular angiotensin I/angiotensin II conversion in patients with chronic heart failure. *Circulation* 101(6)(15 February): 594–97.

Laufs, U., et al. 1998. Upregulation of endothelial nitric oxide synthase by HMG CoA reductase inhibitors. *Circulation* 97(12)(31 March): 1129–35.

Pitt, B., et al. 1999. Aggressive lipid-lowering therapy compared with angioplasty in stable coronary artery disease. *N Engl J Med* 341: 70–76.

Schlaifer, J.D., et al. 1997. Effects of quinapril on coronary blood flow in coronary artery disease patients with endothelial dysfunction. TREND Investigators. Trial on Reversing Endothelial Dysfunction. *Am J Cardiol* 80(12)(15 December): 1594–97.

Yusuf, S., et al. 2000. Effects of an angiotensin-converting-enzyme inhibitor, ramipril, on cardiovascular events in high-risk patients. The Heart Outcomes Prevention Evaluation Study Investigators. *N Engl J Med* 342(3)(20 January): 145–53.

Zannad, F., et al. 2000. Limitation of excessive extracellular matrix turnover may contribute to survival benefit of spironolactone therapy in patients with congestive heart failure: insights from the randomized aldactone evaluation study (RALES). Rales Investigators. *Circulation* 102(22)(28 November): 2700–2706.

Information for Your Doctor about L-Arginine

There are many studies of the effect of L-arginine on endothelial function in humans. The benefit of L-arginine, or lack thereof, depends upon the patient population. Not all forms of endothelial dysfunction benefit from L-arginine administration. Furthermore, L-arginine does not affect endothelial function in healthy people. Intravenous administration acutely restored endothelium-dependent vasodilation in patients with hypercholesterolemia or coronary and peripheral arterial disease. L-arginine also acutely reversed the endothelial dysfunction associated with congestive heart failure, pulmonary hypertension, transplant vasculopathy, tobacco use, Type 2 (but not Type 1) diabetes mellitus, and salt-sensitive hypertension (but not other forms of essential hypertension). The endothelial dysfunction associated with menopause is not improved by L-arginine. However, in postmenopausal women given estrogen, there is an improvement in endothelial function that is further enhanced by L-arginine. There are multiple small double-blind placebo-controlled trials of oral L-arginine, or an arginine-enriched medical food, in patients with cardiovascular disease or risk factors. In patients with coronary artery disease, three of four studies have shown that the addition of L-arginine (6 to 9 grams daily) to standard medical therapy improves endothelial function, treadmill exercise time, and symptoms. However, one study has shown no benefit of L-arginine on endothelial function of the brachial artery in CAD patients with normal endothelial function. In patients with peripheral arterial disease, two of three studies have been positive. Two weeks of L-arginine (8 grams twice daily IV bolus) improved walking distance 76 percent, an effect that was superior to IV prostaglandin therapy. One study using an L-arginine-enriched medical food (6.6 grams L-arginine daily) improved walking distance and quality of life. However, a second study, not yet published at time of writing, showed no significant benefit of the medical food on walking distance or quality of life. In patients with congestive heart failure, two studies have shown that

oral L-arginine improved endothelial function and improved exercise tolerance. There are no studies of L-arginine in primary or secondary prevention.
However, during carotid endarterectomy, intravenous infusion of L-arginine
markedly reduces cerebral microemboli as documented by transcutaneous
Doppler studies of the middle cerebral artery. Side effects of L-arginine are
minimal and infrequent and restricted largely to gastric pain, diarrhea, and
headache. However, like many supplements, there are insufficient data on
long-term safety.

In a recent one-month double-blind, cross-over study in 30 patients with
CAD on appropriate medical therapy, no effect of supplemental L-arginine
was seen on measures of nitric oxide bioactivity and nitric oxide-regulated
markers of inflammation.

References:

Blum, A., et al. 2000. Oral L-arginine in patients with coronary artery disease
on medical management. *Circulation* 101: 2160–64.

Boger, R.H., et al. 1998. Restoring vascular nitric oxide formation by
L-arginine improves the symptoms of intermittent claudication in patients
with peripheral arterial occlusive disease. *J Am Coll Cardiol* 32(5):
1336–44.

Ceremuzynski, I., T. Chamiec, and K. Herbaczynska-Cedro. 1997. Effect of
supplemental oral L-arginine on exercise capacity in patients with stable
angina pectoris. *Am J Cardiol* 80: 331–33.

Clarkson, P., et al. 1996. Oral L-arginine improves endothelium-dependent
dilation in hypercholesterolemic young adults. *J Clin Invest* 97: 1989–94.

Creager, M.A., et al. 1992. L-arginine improves endothelium-dependent vasodilation in hypercholesterolemic humans. *J Clin Invest* 90: 1248–53.

Drexler, H., et al. 1991. Correction of endothelial dysfunction in coronary
microcirculation of hypercholesterolaemic patients by L-arginine. *Lancet*
338: 1546–50.

Lerman, A., et al. 1998. L-term L-arginine supplementation improves small-
vessel coronary endothelial function in humans. *Circulation* 97(21)
(2 June): 2123–25.

Maxwell, A., B. Anderson, and J.P. Cooke. 2000. Nutritional therapy for peripheral arterial disease: A double-blind, placebo-controlled randomized
trial of HeartBar. *Vasc Med* 5: 11–19.

Information for Your Doctor about L-Carnitine

There have been several randomized placebo-controlled clinical trials of
L-carnitine in cardiovascular disease. In 200 patients with symptomatic
CAD, 2 grams L-carnitine daily for 6 months increased exercise tolerance,
reduced ST segment depression with exercise, and improved symptoms. In
a 12-month study of 472 patients post myocardial infarction, L-carnitine
6 grams daily reduced ventricular enlargement. In a 12-month study of 160
patients, 6 grams L-carnitine reduced anginal attacks and was associated
with a survival benefit (1.2 percent versus 12.5 percent mortality, L-carnitine

versus placebo). In 245 patients with peripheral arterial disease, propionyl-L-carnitine 2 grams daily improved walking distance (73 percent versus 46 percent, PLC versus placebo). In 50 patients with CHF, PLC 1.5 grams daily improved walking distance (1.4 minutes versus 0.36 minutes, PLC versus placebo). Significant improvements in maximum exercise times and ejections fractions were reported by Mancini and colleagues in 60 patients with Class II or III CHF randomized either to propionyl-L-carnitine (50 mg tid) or placebo for 180 days (Mancini, 1992). Two other small trials reported similar results. In contrast, the investigators of the Study on Propionyl-L-Carnitine in Chronic Heart Failure (1999) did not show improved exercise tolerance on L-carnitine supplementation.

References:

Brevetti, G., et al. 1995. Propionyl-L-carnitine in intermittent claudication: Double-blind, placebo-controlled, dose-titration, multi-center study. *J Am Coll Cardiol* 26(6): 1411–16.

Cacciatore, L., et al. 1991. The therapeutic effect of L-carnitine in patients with exercise-induced stable angina: A controlled study. *Drugs Exp Clin Res* 17(4): 225–35.

Caponnetto, S., et al. 1994. Efficacy of L-propionyl carnitine treatment in patients with left ventricular dysfunction. *Eur Heart J* 15(9): 1267–73.

Davini, P., et al. 1992. Controlled study on L-carnitine therapeutic efficacy in post-infarction. *Drugs Exp Clin Res* 18(8): 355–65.

Hiatt, W. R., et al. 2001. Propionyl-L-carnitine improves exercise performance and functional status in patients with claudication. *Am J Med* 110(8) (1 June): 616–22.

Iliceto, S., et al. 1995. Effect of L-carnitine administration on left ventricular remodeling after acute anterior myocardial infarction: The L-carnitine echocardiografia digitalizzata infarto miocardico (CEDIM) trial. *J Am Coll Cardiol* 26(2): 380–87.

Mancini, M., et al. 1992. Controlled study on the therapeutic efficacy of propionyl-L-carnitine in patients with congestive heart failure. *Arzneimittelforschung.* (42): 1101–4.

Information for Your Doctor about Coenzyme Q10

The most compelling data for the use of coenzyme Q10 is as adjunctive therapy for patients with congestive heart failure (CHF). CoQ10 also has antioxidant activity and reduces lipid peroxidation, but there is no evidence that it slows the progression of atherosclerosis in humans. The majority of placebo-controlled randomized clinical trials have been positive in CHF, with improvements in NYHA class and fewer hospitalizations for worsening CHF, using doses of 30 to 150 milligrams daily.

In contrast to the positive studies listed, Khatta et al. *(Ann Intern. Med.* 2000) enrolled 55 NYHA Class II–IV CHF patients into a randomized, double-blind, placebo-controlled trial who received 200 mg CoQ10 per day for six months. No differences were documented between placebo and CoQ10 groups for indices of left ventricular ejection fraction, maximal oxygen consumption, or exercise duration.

References:

Bargossi, A.M., et al. 1994. Exogenous CoQ10 supplementation prevents plasma ubiquinone reduction induced by HMG-CoA reductase inhibitors. *Mol Aspects Med* 15(Suppl): S187–93.

Folkers, K. 1985. Basic chemical research on coenzyme Q10 and integrated clinical research on therapy of disease. In *Coenzyme Q*, edited by G. Lenaz. John Wiley and Sons.

Hofman-Bang, C. 1992. Coenzyme Q10 as an adjunctive treatment of congestive heart failure. *J Am Coll Cardiol* 19: 216A.

Morisco, C., et al. 1993. Effect of coenzyme Q10 therapy in patients with congestive heart failure: A long-term multicenter randomized study. *Clin Invest* 71(Suppl 8): S134–36.

Mortenson, S.A. 1990. Coenzyme Q10: Clinical benefits with biochemical correlates suggesting a scientific breakthrough in the management of chronic heart failure. *Int J Tissue React* 12(3): 155–62.

Permanetter, B. et al. 1992. Ubiquinone (coenzyme Q10) in the long-term treatment of idiopathic dilated cardiomyopathy. *Eur Heart J* 13(11): 1528–33.

Weber, C., et al. 1994. Antioxidative effect of dietary coenzyme Q10 in human blood plasma. *Int J Vitam Nutr Res* 64(4): 311–15.

Information for Your Doctor about Chromium Picolinate

Chromium forms a complex with nicotinic acid known as glucose tolerance factor, which appears to be necessary to the action of insulin. Severe chromium deficiency, as has been seen during total parenteral nutrition, is associated with elevated glucose, insulin, and lipid levels as well as CNS disturbance and peripheral neuropathy. Milder chromium deficiency has been purported to be a cause of insulin resistance. There have been several randomized placebo-controlled clinical trials of chromium supplementation, some of which have shown improvements in glucose tolerance in patients with insulin resistance and in diabetes mellitus. However, a systematic review of the literature commissioned by the Office of Dietary Supplements at the National Institutes of Health suggested that there is no effect of chromium supplementation in nondiabetic individuals. In addition, this meta-analysis suggested that the data regarding the usefulness of chromium supplementation for Type II diabetics are not very strong. If chromium supplement is used in a diabetic, assess the response to therapy using markers of glucose tolerance (e.g., plasma insulin, glycosylated hemoglobin, insulin requirements). Side effects are rare. There are case reports of hemolysis and hepatic and renal toxicity in patients consuming over 1,000 micrograms daily.

References:

Althius, M.D., et al. 2001. Dietary chromium supplements and glucose and insulin response: the results of a meta-analysis. *FASEB Journal.* 15(5)(March): A969.

Abraham, A.S., et al. 1992. The effects of chromium supplementation on serum glucose and lipids in patients with and without non-insulin-dependent diabetes. *Metabolism* 41(7): 768–71.

Anderson, R.A., et al. 1993. Chromium supplementation of human subjects: Effects on glucose, insulin and lipid variables. *Metabolism* 32(9): 894–99.

Anderson, R.A., et al. 1997. Elevated intakes of supplemental chromium improve glucose and insulin variables in individuals with type 2 diabetes. *Diabetes* 46(11): 1786–91.

Anderson, R.A., et al. 1991. Supplemental chromium effects on glucose, insulin, glucagon, and urinary chromium losses in subjects consuming controlled low-chromium diets. *Am J Clin Nutr* 54(5): 909–16.

Mertz, W. 1993. Chromium in human nutrition: A review. *J Nutr* 123(4): 626–33.

Uusitupa, M.I. 1992. Chromium supplementation in impaired glucose tolerance of elderly: Effects on blood glucose, plasma insulin, C-peptide and lipid levels. *Br J Nutr* 68(1): 209–16.

Wilson, B.E., et al. 1995. Effects of chromium supplementation on fasting insulin level and lipid parameters in healthy, non-obese young subjects. *Diabetes Res Clin Pract* 28(3): 179–84.

Information for Your Doctor about Fish Oil Supplementation

The strongest evidence indicating a beneficial effect of fish intake on CHD came from the Diet and Reinfarction Trial (DART), in which men who were instructed to eat fish after myocardial infarction (MI) had a 29 percent decline in all-cause mortality as compared with those in the placebo group. However, there is no compelling evidence that fish oil *supplements* reduce cardiovascular events. Nevertheless, fish oil supplementation is useful to reduce triglyceride levels, an effect that is pronounced in those with marked hypertriglyceridemia. The triglyceride-lowering effect is not seen with plant sources of n-3 PUFA (i.e., alpha-linolenic acid). Fish oil also inhibits platelet aggregation, improves endothelium-dependent relaxation, decreases systolic blood pressure, and has antithrombotic, anti-inflammatory, and antidysrhythmic effects. Two concerns regarding fish oil supplementation have been the effect on glycemic control and the ability to reduce triglycerides but slightly elevate LDL-C. More recent data indicate that stable fish oil preparations improve triglycerides and do not adversely effect glycemic control in diabetics. Furthermore, the combination of garlic supplementation with fish oil has a beneficial effect on both LDL-C and triglycerides.

References:

Adler, A.J., and B.J. Holub. 1997. Effect of garlic and fish-oil supplementation on serum lipid and lipoprotein concentrations in hypercholesterolemic men. *Am J Clin Nutr* 65 (February): 445.

De Lorgeril, M., et al. 1994. Mediterranean alpha-linolenic acid-rich diet in secondary prevention of coronary heart disease. *Lancet* 343: 1454–59.

Dietary supplementation with n-3 polyunsaturated fatty acids and vitamin E after myocardial infarction: results of the GISSI-Prevenzione trial. 1999. Gruppo Italiano per lo Studio della Sopravvivenza nell'Infarto miocardico. *Lancet.* 354: 447–55.

Eritsland, J., et al. 1996. Effect of dietary supplementation with n-3 fatty acids on coronary artery bypass graft patency. *Am J Cardiol* 77: 31–36.

Guallar, E., et al. 1995. A prospective study of plasma fish oil levels and incidence of myocardial infarction in U.S. male physicians. *J Am Coll Cardiol* 25: 387–94.

Haglund, O., et al. 1990. Effects of a new fluid fish oil concentrate, Eskimo-3, on triglycerides, cholesterol, fibrinogen and blood pressure. *J Int Med* 227: 347–53.

Kris-Etherton, P.M., T.D. Etherton, and S. Yu. 1997. Efficacy of multiple dietary therapies in reducing cardiovascular risk factors. *Am J Clin Nutr* 65 (February): 560.

Kromhout, D., E.B. Bosschieter, and C. de Lezenne Coulander. 1985. The inverse relation between fish consumption and 20-year mortality from coronary heart disease. *N Engl J Med* 312: 1205–9.

Leaf, A., et al. 1994. Do fish oils prevent restenosis after coronary angioplasty? *Circulation* 90: 2248–57.

McVeigh, G.E., et al. 1994. Fish oil improves arterial compliance in non-insulin-dependent diabetes mellitus. *Arterioscler Thromb* 14: 1425–29.

Meydani, S.N., et al. 1993. Immunologic effects of a National Cholesterol Education Panel step-2 diet. *J Clin Invest* 92: 105–13.

Sacks, E.M., et al. 1995. Controlled trial of fish oil for regression of human coronary atherosclerosis: HARP Research Group. *J Am Coll Cardiol* 25: 1492–98.

von Schacky, C., et al. 1999. The effect of dietary omega-3 fatty acids on coronary atherosclerosis. A randomized, double-blind, placebo-controlled trial. *Ann Intern Med* 30: 554–62.

Information for Your Doctor about Garlic

Two recent meta-analyses of the available trials indicate that garlic preparations reduce total cholesterol by 9 to 12 percent. There has been a range of results, with positive and negative trials, possibly reflecting differences in garlic preparations. A recent meta-analysis suggests that garlic may also have a mild antihypertensive effect, with an average reduction of 7.7/5 mmHg greater than placebo. This effect, and the antiplatelet effect of garlic, may be due to its activation of NO synthase. Because of its antiplatelet effects, garlic could be an additive to other antiplatelet or antithrombotic medications, and potentially increase the risk of bleeding.

References:

Adler, A. J., et al. 1997. Effect of garlic and fish-oil supplementation on serum lipid and lipoprotein concentrations in hypercholesterolemic men. *Am J Clin Nutr* 65: 445–50.

Bratman, S., and D. Kroll. 1999. *Clinical Evaluation of Medicinal Herbs and Other Therapeutic Natural Products,* Rocklin, CA: Prima Publishing.

Das, I., et al. 1995. Potent activation of nitric oxide synthase by garlic: A basis for its therapeutic applications. *Curr Med Res Opin* 13: 257–63.

De Santos, O.S., et al. 1995. Effects of garlic powder and garlic oil preparations on blood lipids, blood pressure and well-being. *Br J Clin Res* 6: 91–100.

Kiesewetter, H., et al. 1991. Effect of garlic on thrombocyte aggregation, microcirculation and other risk factors. *Int J Clin Pharmacol Ther Toxicol* 29: 151–55.

Neil, H.A., et al. 1996. Garlic powder in the treatment of moderate hyperlipidaemia: A controlled trial and meta-analysis. *J R Coll Physicians Lond* 30(4): 329–34.

Silagy, C.A., et al. 1994. A meta-analysis of the effect of garlic on blood pressure. *J Hypertens* 12(4): 463–68.

Steinmetz, K.A., et al. 1994. Vegetables, fruit and colon cancer in the Iowa Women's Health Study. *Am J Epidemiol* 139(1): 1–15.

Warshafski, S., et al. 1993. Effect of garlic on total serum cholesterol: A meta-analysis. *Ann Intern Med* 119(Suppl 7 Part I): 599–605.

Information for Your Doctor about Ginkgo Biloba

Ginkgo biloba extract is a mixture of compounds containing three major groups of substances: 24 percent as flavonoid glycosides, approximately 7 percent proanthocyanides, and 6 percent as terpenoids (DeFeudis, 1991). Four placebo-controlled, double-blind studies have been reported in patients with PAD. A study from Denmark showed no effect in a small group (18 patients) studied for only three months, and used the lowest dose of any of the four studies (120 milligrams daily). The Baur study from Germany randomized 80 patients with stage II PAD for a combination of walking therapy and 120 milligrams daily of EGb 761 or placebo for six months. There was a significantly greater increase (60 percent) in pain-free walking distance in the EGb group (Bauer, 1994). Another study in 33 patients with Fontaine stage IIb PAD was carried out in Germany (Bulling, 1994). The treatment was a walking program, as with the Bauer study, and placebo or a larger dose of EGb 761, 160 milligrams daily, for six months. Both groups more than improved their pain-free walking distances, but the ginkgo group's increase was significantly greater (60 percent). No side effects were attributed to EGb 761 in any of these three studies. In a study of 20 patients with PAD, EGb 761 (320 milligrams daily) was given for four weeks and a significant increase in transcutaneous partial pressure of oxygen (Tc PO_2) was demonstrated in the lower extremities (a 38 percent increase). One controlled clinical trial has reported benefit derived from three months of EGb 761 (160 mg/day) in patients with chronic venous ulcers (Maillet et al., 1994). The mechanism of action of ginkgo has been variously attributed to its antioxidant properties; its enhancement of NO activity; inhibition of platelet-activating factor (Yan et al., 1995; Périanin et al., 1998; August et al., 1994).

References:

Auguet, M., et al. 1994. Ginkgo biloba extract (EGb 761) and the regulation of vascular tone. In *Advances in Ginkgo Biloba Extract Research. Vol. 3. Cardiovascular Effects of Ginkgo Biloba Extract (EGb 761)*, edited by F. Clostre and F.V. DeFeudis. Paris: Elsevier.

Bauer, U. 1994. Ginkgo biloba extact, EGb 761, and its effects on the arteries of the leg. In *Advances in Ginkgo Biloba Extract Research. Vol. 3. Cardiovascular Effects of Ginkgo Biloba Extract (EGb 761)*, edited by F. Clostre and F.V. DeFeudis. Paris: Elsevier. 121–33.

Bulling B. 1994. The treatment of peripheral arterial occlusive disease with walking (blood vessel) training and Ginkgo biloba extract (EGb 761). In *Advances in Ginkgo Biloba Extract Research. Vol. 3. Cardiovascular Effects of Ginkgo Biloba Extract (EGb 761)*, edited by F. Clostre and F.V. DeFeudis. Paris: Elsevier. 143–50.

DeFeudis, F.V. 1991. *Ginkgo Biloba Extract (EGb 761): Pharmacological Activities and Clinical Applications.* Paris: Elsevier.

Maillet, P., et al. 1994. Ginkgo biloba extract (EGb 761) and trophic disorders of the lower limbs: Contribution of EGb 761's anti-ischemic action associated with local treatment. In *Advances in Ginkgo Biloba Extract Research. Vol. 3. Cardiovascular Effects of Ginkgo Biloba Extract (EGb 761)*, edited by F. Clostre and F.V. DeFeudis. Paris: Elsevier.

Périanin A., et al. 1998. Ginkgolide B (BN 52021) and transductional activities of human polymorphonuclear leukocytes. In *Advances in Ginkgo Biloba Extract Research. Vol. 7, Ginkgo Biloba Extract (EGb 761), Lessons from Cell Biology*, edited by L. Packer and Y. Christen. Paris: Elsevier.

Yan, L.J., M.T. Droy-Lefaix, and L. Packer. 1995. Ginkgo biloba extract (EGb 761) protects human low density lipoproteins against oxidative modification mediated by copper. *Biochem Biophy Res Commun* 212(2): 360–66.

Information for Your Doctor about Grape Seed Extract

Oligomeric proanthocyanidin (OPCs) are the active moiety in grape seed extract. In vitro studies suggest that these are more potent antioxidants than vitamins C or E; furthermore, they have antioxidant activity in lipid and aqueous phases. OPCs increase collagen cross-linking, decrease metalloproteinase activity, and reduce capillary permeability. In Europe, OPCs are used to treat conditions associated with capillary permeability or fragility including venous or lymphatic edema; postsurgical or traumatic edema; diabetic retinopathy, and macular degeneration. They are used as antioxidants, with the intent to slow the progression of atherosclerosis, but there are no human studies to support the latter indication. There have been several double-blind placebo-controlled trials in France showing modest benefit in terms of reduced edema and pain in patients with venous insufficiency or postmastectomy.

References:
Bratman, S., and D. Kroll. 1999. *Clinical Evaluation of Medicinal Herbs and Other Natural Products.* Rocklin, CA: Prima Publishing.
Chang, W.C. et al. 1989. Inhibition of platelet aggregation and arachidonate metabolism in platelets by procyanidins. *Prostaglandins Leukot Essent Fatty Acids* 38: 181–88.
Frankel, E.N., et al. 1993. Inhibition of oxidation of human low-density lipoprotein by phenolic substances in red wine. *Lancet* 341: 454–57.
Hertog, M.G., et al. 1993. Dietary antioxidant flavonoids and risk of coronary heart disease: The Zutphen Elderly Study. *Lancet* 342: 1007–11.
Schulz, V., et al. 1998. *Rational Phytotherapy.* New York: Springer-Verlag.
Tixier, J.M., et al. 1984. Evidence by in vivo and in vitro studies that binding of pycnogenols to elastin affects its rate of degradation by elastases. *Biochem Pharmacol* 33: 3933–39.

Information for Your Doctor about Horse Chestnut Seed Extract

The horse chestnut tree bears a prickly fruit that contains one to three large seeds. The seeds are dried and pulverized, then solubilized in alcohol and water. The resulting solution contains the major active ingredient, escin, in addition to hydroxycoumarins, flavonoids, and tannins, alpha- and beta-sitosterol, and stigmasterol. Horse chestnut seed extract has been used for decades in the treatment of chronic venous insufficiency, varicosities, hemorrhoids, and phlebitis in German- and French-speaking countries, where most of the clinical research on these agents has been conducted.

Chronic venous insufficiency is associated with inflammation and increased venous capillary permeability. Escin inhibits the activity of hyaluronidase and elastase, and thereby reverses the increased capillary permeability that occurs with inflammation. The sterols, alpha- and beta-sitosterol and stigmasterol, also exert anti-inflammatory effects. These actions reverse the capillary leakage and inflammatory infiltrate characteristic of chronic venous insufficiency, and thereby reduce edema and pain. Side effects are minimal and are not more frequent (0.6 percent) than placebo in studies of over 5,000 recipients. Another class of bioflavonoid commonly used in Europe for swelling due to lymphatic or venous disease is represented by hydroxyethylrutoside and troxerutin.

References:

Bougelet, C., et al. 1998. Effect of aescine on hypoxia-induced neutrophil adherence to umbilical vein endothelium. *Eur J Pharmacol* 345(1): 89–95.

Bratman, S., and D. Kroll. 1999. *Clinical Evaluation of Medicinal Herbs and Other Natural Products.* Rocklin, CA: Prima Publishing.

Pittler, M.H., and E. Ernst. 1998. Horse chestnut seed extract for chronic venous insufficiency—a criteria-based systematic review. *Arch Dermatol* 134: 1356–60.

Information for Your Doctor about B Vitamins

Although the B vitamins (folate, B_{12}, and B_6) can reduce homocysteine levels, and thereby improve endothelial function, there are no randomized clinical trials showing that vitamin B supplementation reduces heart attack or stroke. Several trials are under way that will provide an answer to this question. Similarly, there are no randomized clinical trials with high-dose vitamin C in the prevention of heart disease. However, there are data indicating that some individuals may be taking too much vitamin C. Pharmacokinetic studies indicate that 200 milligrams vitamin C daily is enough to saturate tissue receptors. Doses higher than this are excreted in the urine. As little as 1 gram of vitamin C per day can increase urinary oxalate levels, even in those without a history of kidney stones. Although high-dose vitamin C or E can improve endothelial function acutely, the long-term effect of high-dose antioxidant vitamins on endothelial function is not known.

Enthusiasm for high-dose vitamin E has waned with the results of the GISSI and HOPE trials. These large randomized clinical trials have indicated that high-dose vitamin E does not reduce cardiovascular events. Most recently, the HATS trial suggests that antioxidant supplementation may even blunt the beneficial effects of statins on HDL cholesterol.

References:

Chambers, J.C., et al. 1999. Demonstration of rapid onset vascular endothelial dysfunction after hyperhomocysteinemia: An effect reversible with vitamin C therapy. *Circulation* 99: 1156–60.

Levine, M., et al. 1996. Vitamin C pharmacokinetics in healthy volunteers: Evidence for a recommended dietary allowance. *Proc Natl Acad Sci USA* 93: 3704–9.

Taddei, S., et al. 1998. Vitamin C improves endothelium-dependent vasodilation by restoring nitric oxide activity in essential hypertension. *Circulation* 97: 2222–29.

Information for Your Doctor about Plant-Derived Sterols

In the early 1950s, Farquhar and colleagues observed that plant-derived sterols decreased serum cholesterol levels. The resurgence of interest in plant-derived sterols is now coupled with the incorporation of these compounds into fat-containing foods. Recently, the FDA has authorized health claims for reduction of cholesterol by products containing plant sterol or plant stanol esters. Plant sterol esters and plant stanol esters may reduce the risk of CHD. Scientific studies show that 1.3 grams per day of plant sterol esters or 3.4 grams per day of plant stanol esters in the diet are needed to show a significant cholesterol-lowering effect (about 10 to 15 percent reduction). Sterols are an essential constituent of cell membranes in animals and plants. Cholesterol is the sterol of mammalian cells, whereas phytosterols produced by plants include sitosterol, campesterol, and stigmasterol. Plant sterols are structurally similar to cholesterol, but are not synthesized by the human body and differ structurally from cholesterol by a methyl or ethyl group in their side chains. These structural differences cause them to be poorly absorbed by the human intestine. They also associate with cholesterol and bile salts to increase cholesterol excretion.

The specific plant sterols that are currently incorporated into medical foods (i.e., Benecol and Take Control) are extracted from soybean oil or pine tree oil. For the most part, the consumption of 2 grams daily of plant sterol ester decreases LDL cholesterol levels 10 to 20 percent. Few adverse effects have been reported with the short-term or long-term consumption of the plant stanol/sterol ester–containing fats. However, of concern are some observations of decreased levels of plasma alpha- and beta-carotene, tocopherol, and/or lycopene and perhaps other fat-soluble vitamins over long periods of time. Until long-term studies are performed to ensure the absence of adverse effects, these products should be reserved for adults requiring lowering of total and LDL cholesterol levels because of hypercholesterolemia or the need for secondary prevention of vascular events.

References:

Blair, S.N., et al. 2000. Incremental reduction of serum total cholesterol and low density lipoprotein cholesterol with the addition of plant stanol ester-containing spread to statin therapy. *Am J Cardiol* 86: 46–52.

Farquhar, J.W., R.E. Smith, and M.E. Dempsey. 1956. The effect of beta sitosterol on the serum lipids of young men with arteriosclerotic heart disease. *Circulation* 14: 77–82.

Miettinen, T.A., et al. 1995. Reduction of serum cholesterol with sitostanol-ester margarine in a mildly hypercholesterolemic population. *N Engl J Med* 333: 1308–12.

Information for Your Doctor about Cardia Salt

Two unpublished randomized clinical trials have supported an antihypertensive effect of Cardia Salt. A double-blind, placebo-controlled clinical study of 223 treated hypertensive patients found that substitution of Cardia Salt for regular salt in the diet and at the table over a six-week period reduced systolic blood pressure by 4 mmHg and diastolic blood pressure by 2.5 mmHg. In another double-blind, placebo-controlled clinical study in 63 hypertensive patients, the substitution of Cardia Salt for table salt over a six-week period reduced systolic blood pressure by 2.5 mmHg and diastolic blood pressure by 5 mmHg.

Information for Your Doctor about the HeartBar

In an open-label dose-ranging study of 41 middle-aged hypercholesterolemic patients, HeartBar improved flow-medicated endothelium-dependent vasodilation in the brachial artery, with a maximal effect at 2 bars daily. In a subsequent double-blind randomized clinical trial, in middle-aged hypercholesterolemic subjects (n = 43), active bar (2 per day) improved endothelial function (by 35 percent), whereas placebo did not change (−3 percent). In one double-blind, placebo-controlled trial study, 41 patients with stage II PAD were randomized to three groups (2 active bars, 1 active and 1 placebo bar, and 2 placebo bars per day), followed by an 8-week open-label period. After 2 weeks of treatment, pain-free walking distance increased 66 percent while total walking distance increased 23 percent in the group taking 2 active bars per day. Quality of life was improved as assessed by SF-36. Significant effects were not observed in the 1 active bar per day and placebo groups. The beneficial effects of two active bars a day were maintained after 10 weeks and, in addition, there was improvement in walking distance observed in the group taking 1 active bar. However, in a subsequent multicenter study (n = 81, unpublished observations) carried out over 12 weeks, there was no significant difference between active and placebo treated groups; each group improved significantly over baseline. The bar has also been studied in patients with CAD. In a randomized, double-blind, placebo-controlled crossover study with 2-week treatment periods separated by a month-long washout period, patients with class II and III angina (n = 36) received either 2 active bars or 2 placebo bars per day. The arginine bar normalized endothelium-dependent vasodilation, whereas placebo had no effect. In addition, the bar significantly increased treadmill exercise time (by 23 percent) and treadmill work (by 33 percent) over placebo, although there was no effect on electrocardiographic measures of ischemia or time to onset of angina. Nevertheless, there was an improvement in quality of life as measured by both the SF-36 and the Seattle Angina Questionnaire. Endothelial dysfunction in hypercholesterolemia is reversed by a nutritional product designed to enhance nitric oxide activity.

References:

Maxwell, A., B. Anderson, and J.P. Cooke. 2000. *Cardiovascular Drugs and Therapy.* June; 14(3): 309–16.

Maxwell, A., et al. 2000. Nutritional therapy for peripheral arterial disease: A double-blind, placebo-controlled randomized trial of HeartBar. *Vasc Med* 5, 1: 11–20.

Maxwell, A.J., et al. 2002. Randomized clinical trial of a medical food for the dietary management of chronic, stable angina. *J Am Coll Cardiol.* Jan. 2; 39(1): 37–45.

Information for Your Doctor about Red Yeast Rice

It is not generally recognized in the medical community that our most powerful antilipid drug is derived from ancient Chinese medicine. In 1979, Endo and colleagues discovered that the strain of Monascus yeast used in the production of red yeast rice elaborates a substance that inhibits cholesterol synthesis. This substance, which he named monacolin K, also known as lovastatin, is known to the medical community as Mevacor. In addition to lovastatin, red yeast rice also contains eight other monacolin-related substances with the ability to inhibit HMG-CoA reductase. Furthermore, red yeast rice contains other agents that may have favorable effects on the lipid levels, including sterols (beta-sitosterol, campesterol, stigmasterol, and sapogenin), isoflavones and isoflavone glycosides, and monounsaturated fatty acids. However, the amount per volume of monacolin K in red yeast rice is small (2.5 milligrams per capsule of statins) when compared to the amount of statin contained in prescription drugs. Therefore, the other ingredients in red yeast rice, such as sterols, may also contribute to lowering cholesterol.

The cholesterol-lowering effects of a proprietary Chinese red yeast rice supplement was studied in hypercholesterolemic patients (n = 83) in a randomized 12-week controlled trial at UCLA. All patients also consumed an American Heart Association Step I diet. In comparison to subjects given placebo, those treated with red yeast rice (2.4 milligrams daily) manifested 17 percent, 22 percent, and 11 percent declines respectively in total cholesterol, LDL-C, and triglycerides.

References:

Heber, D., et al. 2001. An analysis of nine proprietary Chinese red yeast rice dietary supplements: Implications of variability in chemical profile and contents. *J Altern Complement Med* 7: 133–39.

Heber, D., et al. 1999. Cholesterol-lowering effects of a proprietary Chinese red-yeast-rice dietary supplement. *Am J Clin Nutr* 69: 231–36.

Wang, J., et al. 1997. Multicenter clinical trial of the serum lipid-lowering effects of a Monascus purpureus (red yeast) rice preparation from traditional Chinese medicine. *Curr Ther Res* 58: 964–77.

Information for Your Doctor about Selenium

Selenium is required for the activity of the antioxidant enzyme glutathione peroxidase. Selenium deficiency, as in some regions of China, is associated with cancer and cardiomyopathy. Selenium replacement appears to reduce the prevalence of these disorders. A recent double-blind, placebo-controlled randomized trial involving over 1,300 seniors followed for six years demonstrated that in comparison to placebo, selenium (200 micrograms daily) reduced cancer deaths by 50 percent and reduced overall mortality by 17 percent. Epidemiological data is conflicting regarding a relationship between selenium status and cardiovascular mortality. Long-term use of 200 micrograms per day is safe; toxicity is observed with doses over

750 micrograms per day, manifested by GI distress, garliclike odor, hair and fingernail loss, and alterations in mental states.

References:

Clark, L.C., et al. 1996. Effects of selenium supplementation for cancer prevention in patients with carcinoma of the skin: A randomized controlled trial. Nutritional Prevention of Cancer Study Group. *JAMA* 276(24): 1957–63.

Kagan, V.E., et al. 1992. Dihydrolipoic acid—a universal antioxidant both in the membrane and in the aqueous phase. *Biochem Pharmacol* 44: 1637–49.

Neve, J. 1996. Selenium as a risk factor for cardiovascular diseases. *J Cardiovasc Risk* 3(1): 42–47.

Packer, L., et al. 1997. Neuroprotection by the metabolic antioxidant alpha-lipoic acid. *Free Radic Biol Med* 22(1–2): 359–78.

Ziegler, D., et al. 1995. Treatment of symptomatic diabetic peripheral neuropathy with the antioxidant alpha-lipoic acid: A 3 week randomized controlled trial (ALADIN study). *Diabetologia* 38: 1425–33.

Information for Your Doctor about Ribose

Ribose is the sugar moiety of nucleotides, including ATP. Intravenous infusions of ribose have been used to enhance detection of hibernating myocardium conjunction with thallium imaging or dobutamine stress echocardiography. In a small randomized clinical trial, 60 grams of ribose daily for 3 days increased treadmill exercise time to 1 millimeter ST-segment depression by 24 percent.

Information for Your Doctor about Hawthorn

Hawthorn has positive inotropic activity with a broad therapeutic range, antiarrhythmic effects, and can be safely used with diuretics or in patients with renal impairment. In one study, its therapeutic benefit with respect to exercise tolerance in mild CHF was equivalent to 37.5 milligrams of captopril daily. Based on over a dozen clinical trials in Europe, Germany's Commission E approved the use of hawthorn for mild heart failure. It is very well tolerated, and in clinical trials only mild GI distress or allergic reaction was reported. The extract contains a number of agents that may be active, including procyanidins, catechins, flavonoids, purine derivatives, amines, triterpenoids, and aromatic carboxylic acids. It has been found to have activity as a potassium channel activator, cAMP phosphodiesterase inhibitor, angiotensin converting enzyme inhibitor, and an antioxidant.

References:

Bahourn, T., et al. 1994. Antioxidant activities of Crataegus monogyna extracts. *Planta Med* 60(4): 323–28.

Bratman, S., and D. Kroll. 1999. *Clinical Evaluation of Medicinal Herbs and Other Natural Products.* Rocklin, CA: Prima Publishing.

Schulz, V., et al. 1998. *Rational Phytotherapy*. New York: Springer-Verlag.

Seigel, G., et al. Molecular physiological effector mechanisms of hawthorn extract in cardiac papillary muscle and coronary vascular smooth muscle. *Phytother Res* 10: 195–98.

Uchida, S., et al. 1987. Inhibitory effects of condensed tannins on angiotensin converting enzyme. *Jpn J Pharmacol* 43: 242–46.

Information for Your Doctor about Chinese Licorice

Chinese licorice contains glycyrrhizic acid, a mineralocorticoid. This agent increases renal excretion of potassium, and the ensuing hypokalemia can cause ventricular arrhythmias and cardiomyopathy. Chinese licorice antagonizes the action of spironolactone. It is contraindicated in patients with cardiovascular disease.

Information for Your Doctor about St. John's Wort

St. John's wort induces P450 3A4 reductase, and thereby increases the metabolism of many drugs, including cyclosporine. Accordingly, patients using St. John's wort should be warned about drug interactions. There are case reports of St. John's wort causing rejection of transplanted organs because it decreased cyclosporine levels.

For medications, the label is an accurate reflection of what is in the bottle. The FDA holds drug manufacturers to very high standards of purity for medicine. Unfortunately, the FDA does not have this control over supplements. The label on the bottle doesn't always reflect what is inside. As explained on page 205, when the Good Housekeeping Institute analyzed six popular brands of St. John's wort supplement, they found an almost twentyfold difference in potency of the supplements.

References:

FDA Health Advisory, February 10, 2000.

Jobst, K.A., et al. 2000. Safety of St. John's wort. *Lancet* 355: 576.

Ruschitzka, F., et al. 2000. Acute heart transplant rejection due to Saint John's wort. *Lancet* 355: 548.

Information for Your Doctor about Yohimbine

Yohimbine is used as an aphrodisiac. It increases blood pressure and antagonizes the action of clonidine. It is contraindicated in patients with cardiovascular disease.

However, Yohimbine-HCI is an FDA-approved drug for the treatment of impotence. Other forms, such as yohimbe bark extracts and yohimbine (drug form), are sold in health food stores and may contain varying amounts of yohimbine as well as other ingredients. (Yohimbe bark is on the German Commission E's list of unapproved herbs.) Side effects of yohimbine include hypertension, anxiety, headache, and GI symptoms. Large doses can cause severe hypotension cardiac arrhythmias, psychotic reactions, skin eruptions, and death. Yohimbine should not be used by the elderly or individuals with hypertension, heart, kidney, or liver disease.

Information for Your Doctor about Other Supplements That May Interact with Blood-Thinning Medications

A number of supplements can potentially increase bleeding in patients on Coumadin or antiplatelet agents, including CoQ10, danshen, devils claw, dong quai, ginseng, green tea, papain, and vitamin E. Others can interact with digoxin, including kyushin, licorice, plantain, uzara root, hawthorn, and ginseng.

References:

Haller, C.A., and N. Benowitz. 2000. Adverse cardiovascular and central nervous system events associated with dietary supplements containing ephedra alkaloids. *N Engl J Med* 343: 1833–38.

Notes

Introduction

1. All statistics are for 1998 from American Heart Association "2001 Heart and Stroke Statistical Update."

Chapter 1

1. Lord Howard Walter Florey, "The Endothelial Cell," *British Medical Journal* 2 (1966): 487–90.

2. Previous to the discovery of NO, scientists had found another substance made by the endothelium that could maintain vessel health. In 1982, Sir John Vane won the Nobel Prize for the discovery of prostacyclin, a molecule that relaxes the vessel and prevents vessel thickening and clot formation.

3. William Wells, Ph.D., et al., "From Explosives to the Gas That Heals," Beyond Discovery, The Path From Research to Human Benefit, A Project of the National Academy of Sciences, 2001.

4. Ferid Murad, *Les Prix Nobel,* 1998. Published by the Nobel Foundation.

5. R. F. Furchgott and J. V. Zawadzki, "The Obligatory Role of Endothelial Cells in the Relaxation of Arterial Smooth Muscle by Acetylcholine," *Nature,* (27 November) 288(5789) (1980): 373–76.

6. Lawrence K. Altman, "Three Americans Share Nobel Prize in Medicine," *New York Times,* October 13, 1998.

7. Altman, *New York Times.*

CHAPTER 2

1. One year earlier, Hibbs and coworkers had found that white blood cells made nitrite and nitrate (breakdown products of NO) from arginine. Later it would be shown by several groups that the endothelium and the white blood cells each made NO from L-arginine using an enzyme called nitric oxide synthase (NOS).

2. I would like to emphasize that L-arginine is not the solution for everybody. Some people don't need L-arginine; they need a different nutritional and/or medical solution to improve their endothelial function. This book is not just about L-arginine. It is about all of the measures you can take to retain or restore endothelial health. I focus on L-arginine here because it was the first nutritional approach that we took toward improving endothelial function. Perhaps the most important aspect of our observation with L-arginine was that our experiments showed for the first time that a nutritional intervention could rapidly restore an important aspect of endothelial health.

CHAPTER 4

1. We repeated an experiment first performed by Dr. Robert Vogel at SUNY and got the same results. He had shown that endothelial function deteriorates after just one high-fat meal at McDonald's.

2. Sachiko T. St. Jeor, et al., "Dietary Protein and Weight Reduction: A Statement for Healthcare Professionals From the Nutrition Committee of the Council on Nutrition, Physical Activity, and Metabolism of the American Heart Association," *Circulation* 104 (2001): 1869–74.

3. H.O. Bang and J. Dyerberg, "The Bleeding Tendency in Greenland Eskimos," *Danish Medical Bulletin* 27(4) (1980): 202–5; and H.O. Bang, J. Dyerberg, and H.M. Sinclair, "The Composition of the Eskimo Food in Northwestern Greenland," *American Journal of Clinical Nutrition* 33 (1980): 2657–61.

4. As reported in the *Journal of Agricultural and Food Chemistry,* September 2001.

5. Adapted from Susan Mitchell, Ph.D., RD, CNS, presentation to the Annual Meeting of the American Overseas Dietetic Association (AODA), a chapter of the American Dictetic Association, Heidelberg, Germany, March 13, 1998.

CHAPTER 6

1. *The Harvard Women's Health Watch,* June 2001.

CHAPTER 10

1. Industry Overview in *Nutrition Business Journal* 4(6) (1999): 1–5.

2. Estimate of dietary supplement use based on research of Dr. David Eisenberg, Harvard School of Public Health.

3. Good Housekeeping Institute, "New Good Housekeeping Institute Study Finds Drastic Discrepancy in Potencies of Popular Herbal Supplement." News release, Consumer Safety Symposium on Dietary Supplements and Herbs, New York City, March 3, 1998.

4. T. Monmaney, "Labels' Potency Claims Often Inaccurate, Analysis Finds; Spot check of products finds widely varying levels of key ingredient. But some firms object to testing method and defend their brands' quality." *Los Angeles Times,* August 31, 1998.

5. C.A. Haller and N. L. Benowitz, "Adverse Cardiovascular and Central Nervous System Events Associated with Dietary Supplements Containing Ephedra Alkaloids," *New England Journal of Medicine* 343 (2000): 1833–38.

6. Underreporting the use of dietary supplements and nonprescription medications among patients undergoing a periodic health examination. Hensrud et al., Mayo Clinic Pro, 1999.

   Your doctor should be interested in the supplements you are taking. There is no justification for a "don't ask, don't tell" policy for nutritional supplements. These supplements may have beneficial as well as adverse effects on your medical condition. They may interact with your medication. Therefore your doctor needs to have this information. Unfortunately, patients do not always communicate their use of supplements to their doctors. Your doctor may be skeptical of the merit of a supplement; this opinion may be appropriate, as long as the decision is based on a careful review of your case and a knowledge of the nutritional literature.

7. Marian C. Cheung et al., "Antioxidant Supplements Block the Response of HDL to Simvastatin-Niacin Therapy in Patients with Coronary Artery Disease and Low HDL," *Arteriosclerosis, Thrombosis, and Vascular Biology* 21 (2001): 1320.

CHAPTER 11

1. Many of the drugs mentioned in this chapter now have generic forms. Generic drugs are drugs whose patents have run out. This means that any manufacturer can make them. We don't often hear much about these drugs because pharmaceutical companies can't afford expensive advertising for them, no matter how effective they are. Some very good drugs have become generic and are not used as much as they should be.

Glossary

Acetylcholine: A substance made by the body. This substance is often released by nerves. It can stimulate the endothelial cells to release nitric oxide.

ADMA (asymmetric dimethylarginine): A modified amino acid that can block the production of NO. Similar in structure to L-arginine, ADMA can fit into the NOS enzyme, but because it has two extra methyl groups, it can't be made into NO.

Angina: Chest heaviness, pressure, or tightness due to narrowings of the heart arteries.

Aorta and pulmonary artery: The main vessels carrying blood out of the heart. The pulmonary artery carries blood to the lungs. The aorta carries blood to the rest of the body.

Blood glucose: Blood sugar. Glucose, the most common sugar made by the body, is different from the table sugar we sprinkle on our cereal in the morning. Table sugar is sucrose (cane sugar). Each molecule of sucrose is composed of one molecule of glucose and one molecule of fructose. Glucose is the most common form of sugar in nature and is used for energy. In plants, the glucose molecules are stored as starch, which is a complex made of many glucose molecules. In animals, glucose is stored in a complex called glycogen.

Body mass index (BMI): A number that reflects your height and weight. If you have the right weight for your height, you have a normal BMI. If you are too heavy for your height, your BMI will be too high.

Bypass surgery: Surgery in which blood is redirected around a blockage in an artery, usually using a vessel taken from another part of the body.

Chemokine: A member of a large group of proteins that have the ability to lure and attract white blood cells. They are involved in the acute and chronic inflammation of atherosclerosis and infectious diseases.

Cofactor: A substance that helps an enzyme to function. Most often, it is necessary for the cofactor to be present in order for the enzyme to be active or to function properly. For example, a substance called tetrahydrobiopterin (also known as BH4) is a cofactor for NO synthase. Without BH4, NO synthase can't make NO (and instead makes superoxide anion).

Coronary heart disease: Narrowings of the heart arteries, causing angina or heart attack.

C-reactive protein (CRP): A protein in the body that increases during the process of inflammation. It has been found to be an indication of blood vessel inflammation and may be a new way to measure risk of cardiovascular disease.

Cyclic GMP: This is a second messenger for NO. The stimulus of NO causes the formation of cyclic GMP inside the cell. Cyclic GMP has many effects inside of cells. In vascular smooth muscle cells, cyclic GMP causes relaxation.

Cytokine: A small protein released by cells that plays a role in cell interaction, triggering inflammation or a response to infection.

DDAH (dimethylarginine dimethylaminohydrolase): An enzyme that breaks down ADMA. If DDAH is reduced or impaired, ADMA accumulates.

Diabetes mellitus: Diabetes is a condition in which blood sugar is too high. It is too high in Type 1 (or juvenile diabetes) because insulin levels are low. (This type of diabetes affects children, and is not common.) Type 2 diabetes affects adults and is due to a reduced effectiveness of insulin in keeping blood sugar low. Type 2 diabetes is similar to Syndrome X in that both conditions are associated with a reduced response to insulin. However, in Syndrome X the person does not yet have high blood sugar levels. (See Syndrome X, below.)

Fibroblasts: Cells that make connective tissue.

Free radicals: Molecules with an unpaired electron. Electrons in molecules do not like to be unpaired. Therefore, these molecules attack other molecules so that they can share their electrons. When free radicals attack cell membranes or proteins, they damage them. (See oxygen-derived free radical, below.)

Heart failure: A condition in which the heart is weak and has reduced ability to pump blood throughout the body.

In vitro: Studies that are done on cells or tissues outside of the body.

Lipoprotein: A combination of lipid (fat) with the protein that carries it in the bloodstream.

Myocarditis: Inflammation of the heart, often due to a viral infection.

NO (nitric oxide): Originally believed to be nothing more than a product of car exhaust, NO plays an important role in many areas of the body, including the cardiovascular system.

NO synthase (NOS): The enzyme that makes nitric oxide. NO synthase is the factory in the blood vessels where nitric oxide is produced. L-arginine is converted to NO when it fits into the NO synthase enzyme.

Oxidation: The process by which free radicals steal electrons from other molecules. In this way, free radicals can change cell membranes and alter or destroy the function of proteins and small molecules such as nitric oxide.

Oxygen-derived free radical: Molecular oxygen that is converted into an active form of oxygen. This is a molecule with an unpaired electron that wants to be paired. Oxygen-derived free radicals are important in cellular defense against germs, but are a double-edged sword since the inappropriate release of these cell poisons can contribute to aging and disease.

Platelets: Particles in the blood that form blood clots. Platelets are similar to little bags of chemicals, containing serotonin or thrombin and other chemicals. When they come in contact with a damaged endothelium, the chemicals cause the blood vessels to constrict and clots to form. If the endothelium is healthy, platelets are exposed to NO, which prevents clots from forming inside the blood vessel.

Proteins: Proteins are made from amino acids. They are needed to build cells and repair tissue and act as scaffolding to hold cells and tissues together. Specialized proteins interact with genes or produce energy. They also form the antibodies that combat infection.

Prostacyclin (PG12): A sister molecule of NO that also causes vessel relaxation.

Second messenger: A substance that has an action inside of a cell in response to a stimulus on the outside of the cell.

Syndrome X: Also known as insulin resistance syndrome or Reaven syndrome. A disorder of the body's metabolism resulting in high blood levels of triglycerides, low HDL (good) cholesterol, high blood pressure, and resistance to the effect of insulin (the body has to produce more insulin to keep the blood sugar in the normal range).

Superoxide anion: One of the free radicals in the body formed in many biological processes.

Triglycerides: A type of fat that is formed from fatty acids.

Thrombus: Blood clot.

Vascular smooth muscle: The muscular wall of blood vessels. This muscle can contract to narrow the vessel and thereby reduce blood flow through the vessel. This muscle can relax to open up the vessel and thereby increase blood flow.

Weak heart: A failing heart that is pumping less blood out into the body.

Index